EMERGENCY MEDICINE

The Medical Student Survival Guide

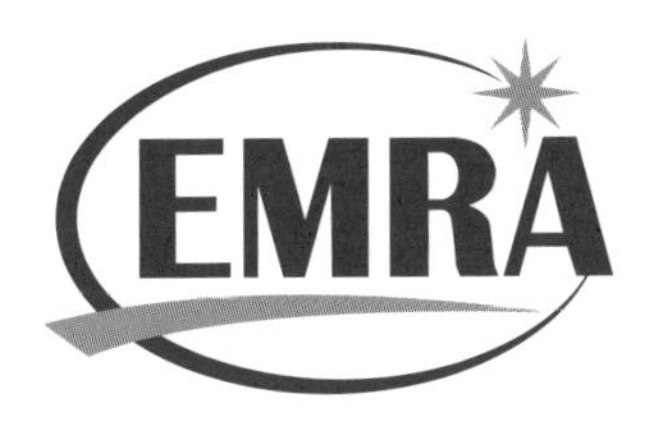

EDITED BY

Joseph Turner, MD, FACEP

David Reid, DO

Dedications

To all the amazing students, residents, and faculty whom I have had the good fortune to work with over the years. You are the reason I have the best job in the world.
— Joe

To my wife, daughter, parents, and entire family for encouraging me to go for my goals, and for picking me up during the inevitable times when some challenges seemed insurmountable. I wouldn't have been able to survive the path through medical school without you! This continues to be a long, hard journey, and I have never taken your support for granted. Thank you!
— Dave

Acknowledgments

We would like to thank all of the members of EMRA without whom this book would not have been possible, including Cathey Wise, Bryan Nyary, and Valerie Hunt. Special thanks to Kristin Harkin, for her guidance as we embarked on this project, and to EMRA Medical Student Council Chair Sean Ochsenbein of ETSU Quillen College and EMRA medical student editor Brian Fromm of the University of Miami, for their contributions throughout the process.

Disclaimer

The Emergency Medicine Residents' Association makes every effort to ensure that contributors to EMRA-sponsored publications are knowledgeable authorities in their fields. Readers are nevertheless advised that statements and opinions expressed in this book are provided as guidelines and should not be construed as EMRA policy unless specifically referred to as such. EMRA disclaims any liability or responsibility of the consequences of any actions taken in reliance on those statements or opinions. The materials contained herein are not intended to establish policy or procedure.

Copyright 2001, 2007, 2012, 2015
Emergency Medicine Residents' Association. All rights reserved.

This book is protected by copyright. No part of this book may be reproduced in any form or by any means without written permission from the copyright holder.

Printed in the USA. ISBN 978-1-929854-41-7.

Additional copies of this publication are available from:
Emergency Medicine Residents' Association
1125 Executive Circle
Irving, TX 75038-2522
972.550.0920
www.emra.org

Editorial Staff

Editors-in-Chief

Joseph Turner, MD, FACEP
Assistant Professor, Emergency Medicine
Indiana University
School of Medicine

David Reid, DO
Emergency Medicine Resident
UT Southwestern/
Parkland Memorial Hospital

Chapter Authors

Michael C. Bond, MD, FACEP, FAAEM
University of Maryland

Carey Chisholm, MD
Indiana University School of Medicine

Jill Corbo, MD, RDMS
Bronx Municipal Hospital Center

Colleen A. Crowe, MD, MPH, FACEP
Medical College of Wisconsin

James Dahle, MD, FACEP
White Coat Investor

Gloria Kuhn, DO, PhD, FACEP
Wayne State University

Jeffrey Manko, MD
NYU Medical Center Emergency Medicine

Amal Mattu, MD, FACEP, FAAEM
University of Maryland

Katie Pettit, MD
Indiana University School of Medicine

Alicia Pilarski, DO
Medical College of Wisconsin

Susan Promes, MD, MBA, FACEP
Penn State Milton S. Hershey Medical Center

Jeremy Sperling, MD, FACEP
New York Presbyterian Hospital

Jonathan St. George, MD
New York Presbyterian Hospital

Tina Sundaram, MD
Albert Einstein College of Medicine

Elizabeth Werley, MD, FACEP
Penn State Milton S. Hershey
Medical Center

Dustin Williams, MD
UT Southwestern /Parkland
Memorial Hospital

Brian Zink, MD, FACEP
Brown University

Online Chapter Authors

Elise Attardo, DO
Christiana Care Health System

Matthew Baird, MD
Steadman Hawkins Clinic of the Carolinas

Whitney Cabey, MD
Carolinas Medical Center

David Cone, MD
Yale University School of Medicine

Myto Duong, MD, MSc
Southern Illinois University

Emily Fitz, MD
Indiana University School of Medicine

Roderick Fontenette, MD, FAAEM
Wright State University,
Boonshoft School of Medicine

Nicolas Forget, MD, MPH, DTMH
Vanderbilt University
Georgetown Public Hospital Corporation

Kendra Grether-Jones, MD
University of California Davis

Camilo E. Gutierrez, MD, FAAEM
Boston University School of Medicine

Melissa Halliday, DO
University of Washington, Division of
Emergency Medicine

Brian Levine, MD, FACEP
Christiana Care Health System

S. Terez Malka, MD
Carolinas Medical Center

Joseph P. Martinez, MD, FACEP, FAAEM
University of Maryland School of Medicine

Lisa Maxwell, MD
Christiana Care Health System

Rakesh D. Mistry, MD, MS
University of Colorado School of Medicine

Josh Mugele, MD
Indiana University School of Medicine

Robert O'Connor, MD, MPH, FACEP
University of Virginia

Scott Schmeissing, MD
Spartanburg Regional Healthcare System

Stephen R. Thom, MD, PhD, FACEP
University of Maryland School of Medicine

Mike Vrablik, DO
University of Washington
School of Medicine

Jennifer Walthall, MD, FACEP
Indiana University School of Medicine

Lindsay Weaver, MD
Indiana University School of Medicine

Michael Winters, MD, FACEP, FAAEM
University of Maryland School of Medicine

2015 EMRA Board of Directors

Matt Rudy, MD
President

Ramnik Dhaliwal, MD, JD
President Elect

Jordan Celeste, MD
Immediate Past President

Alison Smith, MD, MPH
ACEP Representative

David Diller, MD
Academic Affairs Rep

Nathaniel Mann, MD
Secretary/Editor, EM Resident

Anant Patel, DO
Speaker of the Council

Nida Degesys, MD
Vice Speaker of the Council

Jasmeet Dhaliwal, MD, MPH
Legislative Advisor

Leonard Stallings, MD
RRC-EM Representative

Nupur Garg, MD
Informatics Coordinator

Zachary Jarou, MD
Membership Development Coordinator

Sean Ochsenbein, MSIV
Medical Student Council Chair

Ashley Guthrie, DO
Member-at-Large

Welcome to your journey toward becoming an emergency medicine physician! If you have not yet decided on emergency medicine as a career, but instead are simply exploring, that is OK. I would encourage you to learn as much as possible about emergency medicine as there are many misconceptions about the specialty, and it is imperative that you are as informed as possible about choosing the area in which you will spend a 30-year career. If you have not already done so, talk to emergency medicine physicians about their careers, ask about the positives and negatives, and, most important, spend time in the emergency department. And do so as soon as possible! Real-life experience will be your best guide for choosing the specialty that is best for you, but with the Match process coming earlier in recent years, you have a limited amount of time in which to get this experience.

If you have already decided that emergency medicine is right for you, we hope you find this survival guide to be a useful resource on the first step of your journey. The first edition of this book was published in 1991, and over the years Dr. Kristin Harkin and Dr. Jeremy Cushman have provided an invaluable service educating medical students about our specialty. We hope to continue that tradition. This latest print edition has been trimmed down to highlight the most high-yield information from some of the most well-known names in emergency medicine, academicians who have taught hundreds of emergency residents over the years, as well as from a group of bright young stars and leaders in the specialty.

As you work your way through the guide, you may notice a number of topics appear in multiple chapters. This is intentional — these are key points that deserve particular emphasis. On the other hand, there may also be times when advice in one chapter may not line up exactly with advice in another chapter. This is not an accident or oversight. The path from early medical school to residency is not an exact science, and a residency director at one program may have a very different view from the director at another program. Our goal is to draw on opinions from a range of educators at multiple programs to provide you a number of perspectives on issues that are debated amongst emergency medicine leaders across the country.

Because the world of emergency medicine is large and ever-changing, we've prepared supplemental online content that provides additional information for those students who have a particular area of interest (for example, those considering a fellowship).

We hope you find this guide to be useful. This is an exciting time in your life, and we wish you the best of luck.

Joseph Turner, MD, FACEP
Clerkship Director, 4th Year Emergency Medicine Clerkship
Assistant Professor, Department of Emergency Medicine
Indiana University School of Medicine

Want to match into an emergency medicine residency program?

If you're like every other applicant and you've got a ton of questions about how to best prepare yourself for away rotations, ERAS, boards, SLOEs, interviews, and all the other important stuff you need to know, this book can help you get on the right track toward a successful match! There is something for everyone in this Survival Guide, no matter where you go to medical school or where you hope to do your training.

One of the biggest misconceptions about emergency medicine is that everyone who goes into the specialty is the same – that we are all ADD, thrill-seeking, jacks-of-all-trades but masters-of-none. The truth is there are so many different personalities within the EM community. Emergency physicians have a wide variety of interests and expertise in many subjects, in addition to being the best acute care providers in medicine. In the same way, there is no universal advice or path that all EM-minded medical students must follow in order to achieve their goals. Certainly there are gold standards and boxes that have to be checked off along the way, but uniqueness is often appreciated in EM. There are parts of the EM residency application that are different from any other specialty, and residency programs across the country vary greatly in how they view particular attributes of a student's application.

This Survival Guide is a collection of opinions and advice straight from the source! Our authors have been through the process of matching, and many are intensely involved in the review and selection of their programs' residency candidates. EM has become a competitive specialty within the house of medicine. Use this book to identify the strengths and weaknesses of your application. Utilize the advice given to address any concerns about your competitiveness as an applicant. Every effort has been made to generalize the recommendations, but remember, while you may feel like just another number, your situation is unique, and with some hard work, good advice, and a little creativity, you'll find a way to stand out and make programs notice you.

Study hard and get involved. Good luck!

David Reid, DO
Resident
UT Southwestern/Parkland Emergency Medicine Residency Program
Past-Chair, 2014-2015 EMRA Medical Student Council

Table of Contents

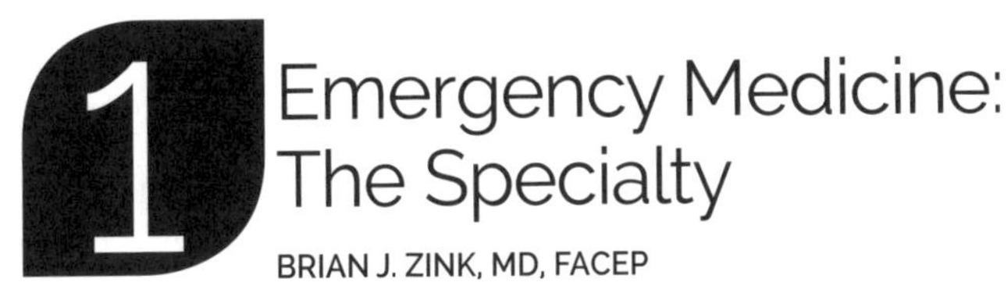

1 Emergency Medicine: The Specialty

BRIAN J. ZINK, MD, FACEP
Professor and Chair
Department of Emergency Medicine
Alpert Medical School, Brown University

In 1961 the Alexandria Hospital emergency room (ER) in Alexandria, Virginia, was reeling from a nearly 300% increase in patient visits in the past decade – up to 18,000 per year. Complaints and wait times were rising. Staffing the ER was a big problem as consigned medical staff objected to working in the ER, and the numbers of house staff had declined by 50%. A plan to use Georgetown University medical students to cover the night shifts had also failed.[1]

> ***The specialty is no longer an afterthought in U.S. health care, but is viewed as a central component of care.***

Into this mix came James Mills, Jr., who had just been made president-elect of the Alexandria Hospital medical staff. Mills, a well-regarded local general practitioner, had worked shifts in the ER, and he liked the pace and variety of cases and was committed to helping the poor and underserved in his community. Mills was also finding his general practice less than satisfying. His idea for solving the problem in the Alexandria Hospital ER was very direct. He put together a plan to contract with the hospital for emergency department (ED) services with himself and three other physicians. These four general practitioners all gave up their private practices and established a contract with Alexandria Hospital for a type of practice that was unheard of in the 1960s. They worked 5 straight days, 12-hour shifts that went from noon to midnight or the reverse. They then had 5 straight days without shifts – an unprecedented schedule in that era.

The Alexandria Plan met some opposition from physicians who could not understand this new type of practice, but it was soon a huge success, with patients and community physicians rallying around the four mavericks. ED visits at Alexandria Hospital doubled in the next 5 years and the physicians were financially viable. The Alexandria Plan garnered a great deal of attention from the world of medicine, the public, the media, and many physicians who wished to replicate it in their own hospitals. Within 5 years a number of Alexandria-type groups had sprung up across the country.

By the end of the decade, emergency physicians began to organize. The first steps were taken in Michigan in 1968 where John Wiegenstein, MD, a tall, statesman-like general practitioner who was working in an Alexandria Plan-like group in Lansing, sought to bring emergency physician colleagues together to develop and deliver educational programs to cover their knowledge and procedural gaps. Another reason for organizing was to push for better reimbursement for emergency care from insurance companies. Wiegenstein collected eight physicians at the Lansing Airport in August 1968, and they decided to come together and boldly called themselves the American College of Emergency Physicians (ACEP). A few months later, a national meeting was held in Virginia that attracted fewer than 40 physicians. A spunky, red-haired physician from Oklahoma, named R. R. Hannas, who had just started practicing emergency medicine but had been involved in gaining specialty status for the field of family practice, explained how a specialty was possible, too, in emergency medicine. He pointed out how a specialty organization like ACEP could be the catalyst to move in this direction, and encouraged the collected physicians to join the Michigan ACEP group. His motion carried, and ACEP was on its way, with John Wiegenstein elected as the first president. ACEP grew exponentially in its first 5 years. The first educational meeting was held in 1969 in Denver, and was audaciously called the "Scientific Assembly." It had little actual science in the meeting proceedings, but it was an important networking venue for the young college.

Most early emergency physicians did not have full training for the type of practice in to which they had migrated. They recognized their deficiencies and realized the field needed more comprehensive residency training in order to create well-rounded practitioners. The first institution to embark on residency training in emergency medicine was the University of Cincinnati, where a young internist named Herb Flessa was assigned to manage the emergency room at Cincinnati General Hospital. Flessa had the pragmatic, but not visionary, idea for a training program to put more bodies in the busy environment where no one else really wanted to work. He applied to the American Medical Association in 1969 and was approved to start a 2-year residency in 1970. The guinea pig for this new residency was Bruce Janiak, MD, who was a Cincinnati medical student with a developing interest in emergency medicine. Janiak basically developed his own 2-year, post-internship residency and became the first emergency medicine resident. His training was largely unsupervised in the emergency department and consisted mainly of various rotations on other services where he did consults and managed patients in the ED. Janiak, as a gregarious person who bonded with people all over the hospital, was successful, and the residency took off, with 5 members in the next class.

Other emergency medicine residencies quickly sprung up at Medical College of Pennsylvania, where pediatric surgeon David Wagner, MD, recruited the first woman trainee in emergency medicine, Pamela Bensen, MD. At the University of Southern California, Los Angeles County Medical Center, OB/gyn Gail Anderson, MD, negotiated to form the first academic department of emergency medicine in 1971. In 1974, the Emergency Medicine Residents' Association (EMRA) was established, and during the next 5 years, more than 30 new emergency medicine (EM) residencies formed.

The early EM residents had to endure constant questioning, second-guessing, and sometimes derision about their career choice. It was pointed out that there was no certifying board in emergency medicine, so they would lack legitimacy in the house of medicine. Despite this, they were highly employable in a wide-open job market. Many EM residency graduates could go directly from training to lucrative positions as medical directors of hospital ED's.

For many of the early residency graduates, who had come of age in the anti-establishment 1960s, having a specialty board in their practice was not a high priority. However, the more senior leaders who had established emergency medicine were determined to gain specialty status. The process was arduous and convoluted. The young field, working through ACEP, had to incorporate as a board, which it did as the American Board of Emergency Medicine (ABEM) in 1976, prepare a certifying examination, and then apply to the American Medical Association (AMA) and American Board of Medical Specialties (ABMS) in a 12-step approval process. The leadership and negotiating team for ABEM consisted of pioneers like James Mills, Jr., John Wiegenstein, and R.R. Hannas, who were more on the practice side, along with Peter Rosen, Gail Anderson, David Wagner, George Podgorny, and Ron Krome, who were more academically oriented. After a year of what they thought was successful hoop-jumping and negotiating, these leaders believed they would be successful in the ABMS delegation vote for ABEM approval. They were very mistaken, as ABMS voted down ABEM 100-5.

The main opposition came from the established boards of internal medicine, surgery, and pediatrics, which questioned whether emergency medicine represented a distinct body of knowledge or specialty practice. But, beyond this more philosophical debate, were concerns about competition for training on ED patients, a fear that medical students would choose emergency medicine over the established disciplines (which was already starting to happen), and loss of revenue as the academic pie would be proportionately smaller with a new member in the mix. Eighteen months of intense, politically charged negotiations ensued, during which the EM leaders compromised by allowing other specialties to have seats on the ABEM board in return for their support. Finally, in September of 1979, the ABMS approved ABEM as a "modified conjoint board," and emergency medicine became the 23rd U.S. medical specialty. The jubilation of the founders of the field was mixed with the realization that a true specialty now needed to emerge, with a strong academic and practice base, a new certifying exam, a residency review process, and active participation in the house of medicine. By 1989, emergency medicine had gained enough of a foothold in the house of medicine to be approved as a primary board by ABMS. In that same year, the Society of Academic Emergency Medicine (SAEM) was formed and became an integral academic presence for the specialty, while ACEP continued to flourish as the largest organized group of emergency medicine physicians. In 1993, the American Academy of Emergency Medicine (AAEM) was formed in an effort to promote the continued ubiquity of residency-trained, board-certified EM physicians in EDs across the country.

The 21st century at the same time, has been a time of tremendous growth in ED utilization by Americans — with more than 136 million ED visits occurring annually by 2012.[2] At the same time, the specialty has matured and has played an important role in shaping health care delivery, advancing the care of acutely ill or injured patients, and leading innovation in medical education. It can be argued that nothing in American medicine has changed as much as emergency care during the past 40 years. In 1970 there were no EM residency programs, and today only internal medicine and pediatrics match more reasidwents than emergency medicine, the National Resident Matching Program.[3] In 1980 there were no board-certified emergency physicians — now there are more than 32,000, according to ABEM records. In 1970 there were no academic departments of emergency medicine — now there are almost 100.

EM research has been focused on clinical care, with a smaller, but very important component of basic science research in resuscitation and cellular injury and ischemia. Many of the improvements in outcomes of patients with acute coronary syndrome, stroke, trauma, sepsis, brain injury, overdose, and other acute conditions can be traced back to pioneering research done by emergency physicians. As in most endeavors in EM, the research teams are almost always multidisciplinary, involving both basic and clinical researchers from other specialties and realms of medicine. In the past few years, EM has become increasingly visible in health care delivery research as we attempt to put science behind our initiatives to improve ED efficiency, patient service and throughput, cost control, and public health.

Education in EM has always been a priority for the specialty. EM led the way in the mid-1980s by becoming the first field to mandate 24-hour attending physician supervision of residents. The innovations of EM in bedside teaching, approaches to didactics, and national educational symposia have been considerable. More recently, academic emergency physicians have played an increasing role in medical student education through EM clerkships or electives, and more generally in curriculum development and positions in the dean's office. For post-residency education, more and more fellowships are available for EM residency graduates.

On a national level, the broad perspectives, multidisciplinary approach, and decisive nature of emergency physicians have propelled many to leadership positions in government, politics, and medical organizations. In 2015, the AMA presidency was filled for the first tie by an emergency physician, Steven Stack, MD, FACEP.

EM is immersed in the day-to-day lives of people and their communities. As such, it is called upon to be both watchdog and rescue dog for emerging crises. Whether it is an infectious epidemic first picked up by ED surveillance, or the mass casualty response to a hurricane, tornado, or terrorist bombing, EM is at the center of detection, planning, and response. This utilitarian role has extended to global health, where U.S. emergency physicians have played key roles in building emergency care capabilities and educational programs in developing nations.

The future of emergency medicine appears to be very bright. The specialty is no longer an afterthought in U.S. health care, but is viewed as a central component of care. Pressure to reduce ED visits and costs may result in less rapid growth in ED visits, but this may be offset by the aging population and increased ability to intervene when patients decompensate. The importance of emergency medicine as a diagnostic center and crossroads of care is increasingly realized. The development of observation units, enhanced case management, and improvements in the interface with home care and skilled nursing facilities all have the potential to improve care and reduce overall costs of care. Rather than being viewed as a place where inappropriate and expensive visits occur, EDs should be utilized as clinical hubs where rapid assessment, treatment, and follow-up care can produce better outcomes and more satisfied patients while saving health care dollars.

Fifty years later, as we reflect on the pioneering physicians who created the Alexandria Plan, organized the specialty, developed the first training programs, and achieved ABMS specialty status for emergency medicine, we confront similar issues but in a very different environment of care. However, the legitimacy and importance of emergency medicine is no longer in question. Our charge now, in this challenging new era of health care reform, is to be as innovative, persevering, and visionary as the founders of the field.

REFERENCES

1. Zink, BJ. Anyone, anything, anytime — a history of emergency medicine. 2006, Mosby Elsevier; Philadelphia, PA.
2. http://www.cdc.gov/nchs/fastats/emergency-department.htm; National Hospital Ambulatory Medical Care Survey, 2011.
3. NRMP match statistics, 2015. http://www.nrmp.org/wp-content/uploads/2015/03/ADT2015_final.pdf

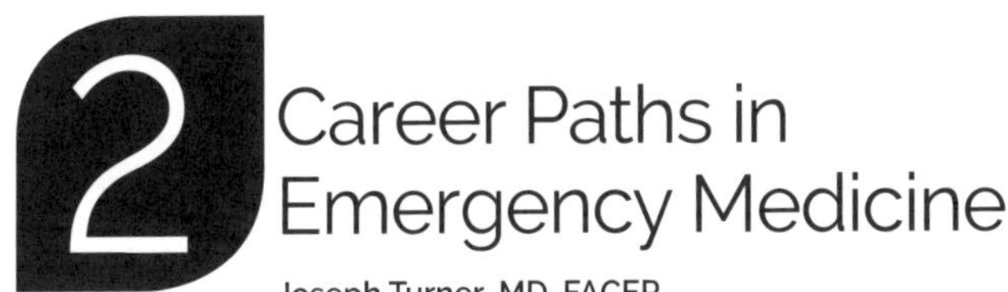

2 Career Paths in Emergency Medicine

Joseph Turner, MD, FACEP
Clerkship Director, 4th Year Emergency Medicine Clerkship
Assistant Professor, Department of Emergency Medicine
Indiana University School of Medicine

Medical students may be drawn to emergency medicine for a variety of reasons. Some may have prior connections to a particular aspect of the specialty such as emergency medical services. More commonly, prospective emergency physicians have broad interests and a diverse skill set, seeing themselves as a jack-of-all-trades. The good news is emergency medicine offers multiple possible career paths for medical professionals with diverse personalities and interests.

> ***The flexibility of emergency medicine will allow you to maintain a rewarding career.***

When discussing potential emergency medicine careers, the first and most substantial distinction is between a career as a community emergency physician and a career in academic practice. As we will discuss, the situation is more complex than this. Within both the community and academic spheres there are multiple different practice patterns and environments. Moreover, the line between community practice and academics is blurred in many settings, with physicians incorporating elements of each into their careers. Other paths also exist. Emergency physicians can maintain careers in the armed forces or practice internationally. ACEP even maintains a section on cruise ship medicine. Additional education may be obtained in the form of other post-graduate degrees (e.g., PhD, JD, MPH, etc.) or fellowship training, opening up new patterns of practice. Emergency medicine can even be combined with other specialties formally recognized by the American Board of Medical Specialties.

This wide variety of possible career paths in emergency medicine is one of the great aspects of the specialty. Whether you have a passion for a specific niche that falls under the scope of emergency medicine, or you are someone who likes to get involved in everything, it is likely that the specialty will be able to accommodate your interests. More important, the flexibility of emergency medicine will allow you to maintain a rewarding career as your personal and professional needs change over time.

Community Practice

The most frequent career path chosen by emergency physicians is commonly known as "community practice." Typically, this refers to a career in which the physician does not hold a formal academic faculty appointment. The term is somewhat misleading, as all emergency physicians, including those working in an academic setting, certainly work as part of a community. Furthermore, non-academic physicians practice in many disparate environments associated with numerous practice patterns; as a result the practice of one "community physician" may look quite different from another. Nevertheless, the term remains in popular use to refer to emergency physicians who do not have a formal academic career.

According to data from the Association of American Medical Colleges (AAMC), 87.8% of the 13,209 emergency physicians who graduated residency from 2004-2013 had no active faculty appointment, and 82.4% had never had a faculty appointment.[1] In other words, the vast majority of emergency physicians practice primarily in the community setting. However, within this vast umbrella, community emergency physicians practice in a myriad of environments, ranging from 5-bed rural emergency departments to massive urban trauma centers that see more than 100,000 patients per year.

Practice patterns within the community setting can vary as much as the practice environment. Many community emergency physicians work for democratic groups. As the name implies, each member of a democratic group has a say in major decisions affecting the group and shares in the group's benefits, as well as their responsibilities. A slight variation on the democratic group is a group that has a partnership track. Groups with partnership tracks reward members who have been part of the group for a designated time period and have made significant contributions by providing them with additional benefits such as an ownership stake or profit sharing, more favorable schedules, and/or greater influence in group decision making. Both democratic groups and partnership track groups are considered a type of private practice. Typically the group enters into an agreement with a hospital or group of hospitals to provide emergency department coverage, but maintains a fair amount of independence regarding their internal affairs. Being a member of a private practice group can be quite appealing, as it offers a sense of freedom and ownership for the emergency physician. At the same time, it comes with added responsibilities and demands, including operating the group's administrative and financial structure and working to maintain good relationships (and frequently renegotiating contracts) with associated hospitals. There is even a risk of potentially losing the contract with the associated hospital.

On the other end of the spectrum, many emergency physicians work strictly as employees of a larger organization, without maintaining a stake in the ownership of that organization. They may work as employees of a contract management group, a corporation that employs a large number of physicians and may hold contracts with numerous hospitals. Physicians also can be employed directly by the hospital, either as a full staff member with benefits or as an independent contractor. These types of arrangements appeal to many physicians, as the contract management group or the hospital will usually handle the bulk of the administrative and billing duties, leaving clinical care as the physician's main responsibility. On the other hand, such practice patterns generally leave individual practitioners less vested in the practice and may be associated with fewer opportunities for advancement and leadership. At the extreme end of this type of work is locum tenens, in which a physician, often in association with a placement agency, fills holes in coverage at multiple hospitals. This type of practice can be associated with significant freedom, the ability to travel, and considerable financial reimbursement, though at the expense of even less investment than the previously mentioned models and decreased job security.

There are both significant rewards and important downsides to a career in community emergency medicine practice. One appealing aspect of this career path is that community practice jobs usually have fewer requirements and demands on time outside of clinical shifts than academic jobs. They also are frequently associated with a higher salary. Most emergency physicians change jobs at some point in their careers, and the larger number of available community positions offers greater flexibility to the physician whose personal and professional needs change over time. Lack of competition from learners offers greater opportunities for community physicians to use and maintain the procedural skills they worked hard to acquire during residency. In many locations, direct interaction between the emergency physician and consultants can promote a sense of camaraderie and investment in the greater hospital community.

On the other hand, community physicians may still have significant demands outside of their clinical responsibilities; in particular, if they are part of a private practice group, they may need to help take care of many administrative and financial tasks. Often, these tasks may require skill sets in which they do not feel adequately trained. Community practice groups may have less secure ties to the hospital and have to continually face the challenges of contract negotiation. Prolonged periods away from an academic center can place a larger burden on the community physician to take the initiative to stay abreast of the latest emergency medicine advances and evidence. Fortunately, the robust resources available to the practicing physician, including those provided by ACEP, SAEM, AAEM, and other national societies, make this much more feasible.

Regardless of the specific practice environment, the majority of those who choose community practice will find it to be a stimulating and rewarding career. It challenges one's clinical skills, while at the same time offering numerous extra-clinical benefits. Most community practice models offer opportunities for leadership and skill advancement beyond medicine. Many, despite not being academic positions, offer the opportunity to teach members from multiple health professions. Finally, they tend to be associated with significant time to pursue outside interests, as well as competitive financial compensation and flexibility in lifestyle.

Academic Practice

Academic practice refers to careers in which the emergency physician holds a formal appointment with an academic teaching center, most frequently an accredited U.S. medical school. As with community practice, there is a wide range of environments in which academic emergency physicians practice, from small community-affiliated hospitals to large county hospitals. Most commonly, however, the academic emergency physician will practice at a tertiary care center associated with learners from multiple different medical specialties. Also like community practice, the group structure and contract models of academic practices can vary considerably.

There are two common career tracks for the academic physician: a tenure track and a clinical track. Tenure tracks follow the traditional model associated with other university academic departments. Faculty members are expected to demonstrate achievement in different areas of focus that vary by institution but frequently include teaching, research, and service. They submit their curriculum vitae and dossier for review in order to obtain promotion to a higher academic rank. After a designated time period, the faculty's performance is reviewed for consideration of tenure, and if the individual does not meet the defined requirements, s/he can lose the academic appointment. It is important to note that specific guidelines for promotion and tenure vary substantially from institution to institution.

Recognizing there are many excellent educators who make significant contributions to medical schools and residencies, but who do not have a particular research interest, most institutions also have a separate track for clinical educators. In this model, faculty are still expected to demonstrate contributions to the university in multiple areas, but the requirements for promotion are adjusted to accommodate the clinical workload. Faculty on these tracks still undergo review for promotion through the academic ranks, and academic achievement may be associated with extension of an offer for a long-term contract.

Like community practice, there are both positive and negative aspects to a career in academics. Many physicians find working with medical students and residents, disseminating knowledge, and shaping future practice to be very rewarding. Interactions with other faculty and learners in an academic setting may be more engaging than those in a community setting. Some individuals find research and the discovery of new knowledge inspiring. Academic departments typically have numerous opportunities for career advancement and leadership, not only within the department but also within associated medical schools and hospitals. They also provide a strong administrative structure and numerous resources that faculty can use to aid their continuing education and professional development.

On the other hand, academic positions are frequently associated with slightly lower salaries than comparable community positions. Fortunately, this is often balanced to some extent by quality benefit packages associated with academic positions. Academic positions also have more extra-clinical demands on the physician's time. Examples include grand rounds or journal club attendance, delivery of didactic presentations, time spent filling out learner evaluations, and production of scholarly material. Again, specific requirements vary widely from institution to institution. Academic physicians may also find they have to sacrifice procedural opportunities to their learners. Finally, the lower number of available academic positions may mean that those seeking those positions cannot limit their search based on geographical considerations.

For those who find aspects of both community practice and academics appealing, opportunities exist for educating medical students and residents without being a member of the core faculty group at an academic institution. In many locations, emergency medicine residents, residents from other specialties, and medical students may all have the opportunity to do rotations in emergency departments not formally affiliated with an academic institution. Physicians practicing in the departments become "quasi-academic" faculty, teaching the learners and possibly even holding volunteer affiliate faculty appointments with the learner's home institution, but without all the other requirements that come from a full faculty appointment at an academic institution.

Emergency Medicine Combined Residency Programs

While the majority of emergency physicians do their clinical work exclusively in the emergency department, other models exist. Emergency physicians can be found practicing medicine in clinics, on the wards, and in the ICU. Typically, this involves additional training to provide the skills necessary to be successful in these areas. Some emergency physicians even become board-certified in a second specialty, and residency training programs currently exist that allow learners to become dual certified in emergency medicine and internal medicine, pediatrics, or family medicine. Several emergency medicine/internal medicine programs also offer a 6-year track that adds critical care training for triple certification.

Fellowships

Fellowships are training programs a physician may elect to enter following completion of his/her emergency medicine residency. They provide specialized training in a specific area of emergency medicine such as emergency medical services, ultrasound, or toxicology. This offers many potential advantages, including making you more marketable for certain positions, especially academic positions, providing structured mentorship, and allowing you to further develop expertise in an area of interest. Of course, this must be balanced against the additional learning demands and the financial impact of losing 1-2 years of salary that a practicing emergency physician would make. This is especially significant, because, unlike other areas of medicine, fellowship training in emergency medicine typically is not associated with higher post-fellowship pay compared with one's peers.

There are two major types of emergency medicine fellowships: those that are recognized by the ABEM and provide the opportunity for formal certification in the subspecialty of choice, and those that do not.

Choosing a Career Path

If you already have an idea of what kind of career path you would like to pursue, great. This will help you identify mentors and tailor your training to your specific interests from the start of residency. On the other hand, if you are unsure what type of career path is right for you, don't fret. Many incoming residents do not know what kind of career they want, and many others change their plans over the course of their residency training. Residency will give you numerous opportunities for exploration, and the great news is that emergency medicine is broad enough to cover most interests.

REFERENCES

1. AAMC survey https://www.aamc.org/data/420832/tablec7.html

For more information about combined specialties and fellowships, please see the Medical Student Survival Guide *online at emra.org.*

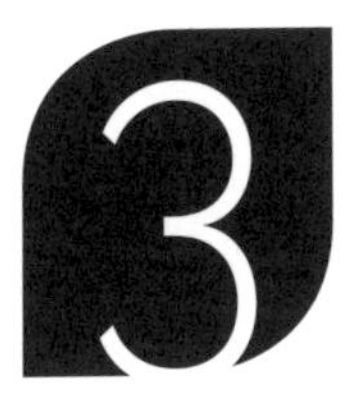

Mentoring in Emergency Medicine

Gloria J. Kuhn, DO, PhD, FACEP
Vice Chair for Academic Affairs
Department of Emergency Medicine
Wayne State University

Medical schools are becoming more aware of the need for and value of mentoring medical students.

When you're a medical student, finding a mentor is extremely important. You are in a new and unknown environment, attempting to make decisions that will affect your future. This can be a very stressful and uncertain period. You might be far from family and friends who could provide support systems, companionship, and advice. During medical school you are faced with learning large quantities of complex information, frequent examinations, and the knowledge that your ability to gain the residency and medical career of your choice is associated with your success in medical school (translate this to good grades and evaluations). Mentors can help you face some of these challenges, and studies have shown that the majority of residents who were mentored as students found it to be very helpful.[1] Figures 1 and 2 highlight some of the ways a mentor can help.

These reasons are why 90-95% of medical students rate mentorship as valuable and want to find a mentor.[2] The mentor can make the difference between floundering for months trying to figure out how to be successful and navigating the system smoothly, with clear goals and help in making decisions that are right for you.[3,4] It is a relationship that may last for many years if both parties give it the attention it needs to flourish. The article by Gillespie offers a wonderful discussion of the responsibilities of each party and is recommended reading for anyone interested in finding or being a mentor.[5] This chapter will provide practical advice on finding a mentor and making the relationship work.

FIGURE 1. VALUE OF HAVING A MENTOR

Receive help in navigating the medical school system and in time management.
Earn better grades and advance further in your careers.
Be introduced to and guided into medicine as a profession.
Have a source for help in choosing and finding elective rotations to further your career.
You'll be more inclined to teach and mentor others.
You'll be more successful in developing strong professional relations.
You'll be more satisfied in your career.

FIGURE 2. ACTIONS OF MENTORS

Help students clarify both short- and long-terms goals and solve problems.
Help the student find a position on a research project.
Assist the student in finding a job or "fellowship" during a summer vacation.
Coach the medical student for interviews, write personal statements, and prepare a curriculum vitae.
Introduce the student to colleagues who can help them in their careers.
Assist the student in getting into the residency of his/her choice, including writing letters of recommendation.

Definition of a Mentor and Types of Mentoring Relationships

My favorite definition of mentor is "a purveyor of dreams," as stated by Peter Rosen, one of the fathers of emergency medicine, during a presentation on mentoring. This statement is so simple and yet so profound. But there are other definitions of mentor that range from a broad explanation of a mentor "... as a person with whom one meets for advice on any topic"[6] to a more narrow definition of "a naturally formed one-to-one relationship between a junior and senior person designed to promote personal and professional development beyond any particular curricular or institutional goals."[7] The terms mentor, adviser, coach, and teacher are often used interchangeably. It is the relationship that determines if someone is a mentor. What is important is not memorizing definitions but realizing the value of finding and having a good mentor and understanding that you must value and nurture the relationship as much as your mentor does. The relationship is dynamic, evolving over time with the roles of mentor and mentee being defined and redefined to fit the needs of both.[3]

Types of Mentoring Programs and Relationships

Medical schools are becoming more aware of the need for and value of mentoring medical students, and many schools have begun formal mentoring programs. These vary in format. Some formal programs assign faculty in either a one-to-one relationship or to a group of medical students. In team mentoring there may be one or a combination of volunteer/assigned faculty and a volunteer junior or senior medical student. By contrast, informal mentoring occurs because a student respects and admires a faculty member and requests mentoring, or a faculty member respects a medical student and offers to be an adviser or mentor. One study found that when students selected their own mentor(s) the relationship felt less forced, more natural, and actually had a better chance of success.[8] In a study of formal mentoring programs for internal medicine residents, 90% chose individual mentoring, supporting the value placed on the relationship.[9,10]

Often students will find a number of advisers/mentors, a model known as mosaic mentoring. The advantage of this model is that different mentors have expertise and experience in various areas of importance, such as a career in a particular specialty or insight into which electives/rotations to choose. For many students this works well; however, be careful not to become confused over conflicting advice. Informal mentoring by junior or senior faculty or by a more senior medical student are all possibilities. Near-peer mentoring is a model in which junior or senior medical students are linked to new medical students in the program. Research on this model showed mentees met more often and did not feel as intimidated as with a senior faculty member who might have some power over them and who they might want to impress. Peers are closer to the problems faced by new students. One study found that medical students benefited socially, academically, and emotionally from this model.[4] Figure 3 compares formal and informal models of mentoring.

FIGURE 3. COMPARISON OF FORMAL AND INFORMAL MENTORING PROGRAMS

Formal Mentoring Programs	Informal Mentoring Programs
Faculty and students are assigned to each other. Participation of the student is usually voluntary. There are often activities planned by the program or mentor for mentees.	The student requests mentoring from one or more faculty they know or have heard about. The relationship is voluntary and lasts as long as both parties find it of value.
Types One-on-One Team Mentoring Near-Peer Mentoring Combination of all of these	**Types** One-on-One Mosaic: The student finds multiple mentors

Frequency of Meetings Set by the program and/the mentor. The student can request a meeting with the mentor if a question or issue arises.	**Frequency of Meetings** The student is usually responsible for requesting meetings. Ideally, the student helps plan the agenda and reports progress on actions suggested by mentor and accepted by the mentee.
Chances for Success This depends on whether the student and mentor can build a relationship that the student finds helpful and that both value. Some of these relationships have continued for many years.	**Chances for Success** The chances are good as the mentor is usually someone the student respects and likes. It is necessary for the mentor to make time available for meetings and take a genuine interest in helping the student.

Choosing a Mentor and Building the Relationship

You and your mentor are equally responsible for a successful relationship.

Authors who have studied mentoring mention the concept of the "chemistry" or "personality fit" between the mentee and the mentor.[11] People pick and choose their friends based on mutual interests and a sense of compatibility. This is true of mentors and mentees as well. At the beginning, the relationship may feel awkward unless you've known your potential mentor for a period of time. Then the issue is simply having the courage to request mentoring. After you identify a potential mentor, set a meeting to ask if s/he has time for and interest in the relationship. That first meeting is really a get-to-know-you period, determining what you want from the relationship and setting expectations such as frequency of meetings and issues to discuss.

Other times the relationship may begin when you request a meeting with a faculty member to ask advice on a subject. Faculty members who are interested in helping will make time for this type of meeting and show interest in your opinions and welfare. This is a particularly good way to find a mentor. It does not commit anyone to the more intense relationship of mentorship but allows you to meet the faculty member privately, ask questions, and determine if there is good chemistry or personality fit. If there is not, then nobody feels awkward about letting the relationship dwindle, but if there is, you can ask about the possibility of some future meetings to get advice. Most faculty members will accept the request, and the relationship will grow. Faculty who work in academic settings enjoy the mentoring relationship and get a sense of fulfillment in helping future colleagues who are entering the profession of medicine.

Personality fit and the relationship are more important than gender concordance.[6] Some students prefer gender concordance for a variety of reasons while others don't care. Successful mentoring relationships are based on reciprocity, respect, clear expectations, and shared values.[12]

Some students feel more comfortable with a mentor of the same race, culture, or ethnicity. If this is the case it should be respected and the student helped to find a suitable mentor, which can often be done using distance mentoring. Mentoring minority students may be especially valuable in helping them integrate into the student body, feel welcome, develop the study habits leading to success in medical school, and be confident that the decisions they are making and actions they are taking are right for them.

Characteristics of a Good Mentor

Good mentors have a number of attributes, as shown in *Figure 4*. If you do not sense these qualities in your mentor, the relationship will not grow, and you may find yourself seeking a mentor better suited to your needs.

FIGURE 4. ATTRIBUTES OF A GOOD MENTOR

Interested in the mentoring relationship, making time for meetings and keeping appointments
Does not attempt to impose his/her opinions on your decisions
Is willing to discuss a broad range of topics of interest to you
Helps you with goal-setting and finding opportunities to further those goals
Good listener who is non-judgmental but will point out pros and cons of your decisions
Is knowledgeable about the institution and the career of medicine
Never attempts to take advantage of you

Being a Successful Mentee

You are equally responsible for making the relationship successful as your mentor. See *Figure 5*. While a meeting with your mentor should be enjoyable, it is also a "working" session to help you discuss and cope with a variety of issues. This means respecting your mentor's time by keeping and being punctual for appointments. If you will be late or forced to cancel an appointment, call and explain the situation. Canceling appointments should be kept to a minimum. Think about the issues you wish to discuss and why before the meeting. This is not a complaint session but rather a time to discuss issues, find solutions for problems, and go over steps in furthering your career. Sometimes you might simply want to say hi and talk to a mentor you have come to regard as a friend. This kind of meeting is very rewarding for the mentor, but you must understand

and respect crowded schedules. Sometimes your mentor may only have time for a very brief "hello," and sometimes you might need to simply ask an administrative assistant to let your mentor know you stopped by.

FIGURE 5. CHARACTERISTICS OF A GOOD MENTEE

Respects time limits (i.e. , making appointments in advance, keeping appointments, ending on time, and informing the mentor if you will be late or need to cancel an appointment)
Prepares an agenda of items to discuss and possible solutions if you have a problem (and admits when you don't know what to do about something)
Listens to advice and is honest about any reasons for rejecting that advice
Suggests a timeline for recommended actions and follows through on it
Drives the relationship by making appointments, listening to advice, and completing actions

Barriers to Mentoring

Mentoring works best when both parties are involved and engaged in the relationship. However, some students are apathetic, even with near-peer mentoring, and others miss out on the benefits of mentoring because they don't know how much it can help, they're too shy to approach a mentor, or they're overwhelmed by schoolwork. Some institutions build time for meetings into the curriculum, helping to foster the mentoring relationship.

If your school does not have formal mentoring programs, faculty can provide advice in a lecture on the value of mentoring and how to find one. If the relationship fails either because the mentor is disinterested or personalities are not compatible, this may inhibit the student from seeking out a different mentor who might prove to be "right" for that student.

Finally, time is a significant barrier, as both you and your mentor have busy schedules. Both must make a commitment to the relationship and feel a sense of value and satisfaction so you each make meetings a priority. Planning ahead for face–to-face meetings, communicating via email, phone, texting, or by Skype are all solutions to the time barrier.

Ending the Relationship

One or both parties may wish to end the relationship. If the mentor ends it, then it is usually due to a move to another institution or a job change. If the relationship has been very successful, the mentor may offer the option of continuing using long-distance methods. You might feel the need to accept. If this solution doesn't work well, the relationship will gradually fade.

Usually it is the mentee who wants to end the association, for any of a variety of reasons. This may be a natural evolution related to graduation from medical school, completion or residency, or a job change that requires moving. Decide if the relationship is still meaningful, and if it is, ask your mentor if you can continue contact via phone, emails, or Skype.

Sometimes a mentee is either uncomfortable with the relationship or feels it is not helpful. A graceful way to end is to make an appointment and thank your mentor for past help, reiterating how it was valuable and has helped you in your career. You have the right to end the relationship at any time and should not feel guilty about this. Sometimes a mentoring relationship fails. This may be due to lack of commitment by one or both parties, lack of communication, poor personality fit, perceived or real competition, and the mentor's lack of experience in mentoring.[12] A good mentor will not be upset and will not cause feelings of guilt.

Summary

Mentoring can be one of the most helpful relationships for medical students, residents, junior faculty, and even senior faculty. It is difficult to see ourselves objectively and having the opportunity to discuss ideas, problems, or a range of issues with a trusted colleague or mentor is extremely helpful and satisfying. Mentors get a sense of satisfaction and even rejuvenation from the relationship. Finding the right mentor will take some time and effort, but it's well worth the work involved for the valuable dividends it will offer. After you realize these benefits as a mentee, act as a mentor to someone, be it a high school or college student contemplating going into medicine, a medical student or resident, or someone coming to you for your advice and help. Always remember, you have a lot to offer should you choose to help - and if you feel you can't help, point them to someone who can.

REFERENCES

1. Frei E, Stamm M, Buddeberg-Fischer, B. Mentoring programs for medical students—a review of the PubMed literature 2000-2008. *BMC Med Educ*, 2010.10:32.
2. Aagaard EM, Hauer KE. A cross-sectional descriptive study of mentoring relationships formed by medical students. *J Gen Intern Med*, 2003. 18(4):298-302.
3. Garmel GM. Mentoring medical students in academic emergency medicine. *Acad Emerg Med*, 2004. 11(12): p. 1351-7.
4. Singh S, Singh N, Dhaliwal U. Near-peer mentoring to complement faculty mentoring of first-year medical students in India. *J Educ Eval Health Prof.* 2014. 11:12.

5. Gillespie SM, et al. Love letters: an anthology of constructive relationship advice shared between junior mentees and their mentors. *J Grad Med Educ*, 2012. 4(3):287-9.
6. Levine RB, et al. "A good career choice for women": female medical students' mentoring experiences: a multi-institutional qualitative study. Acad Med, 2013. 88(4):527-34.
7. Rose GL, Rukstalis MR, Schuckit MA. Informal mentoring between faculty and medical students. *Acad Med*. 2005. 80(4):344-8.
8. Straus SE, Chatur F, Taylor M. Issues in the mentor-mentee relationship in academic medicine: a qualitative study. *Acad Med*, 2009. 84(1):135-9.
9. Levy BD, et al. An initiative in mentoring to promote residents' and faculty members' careers. *Acad Med*, 2004. 79(9):845-50.
10. Yeung M, Nuth J, Stiell IG. Mentoring in emergency medicine: the art and the evidence. *CJEM*, 2010. 12(2):143-9.
11. Jackson VA, et al. "Having the right chemistry": a qualitative study of mentoring in academic medicine. *Acad Med*, 2003. 78(3):328-34.
12. Straus SE, et al. Characteristics of successful and failed mentoring relationships: a qualitative study across two academic health centers. *Acad Med*, 2013. 88(1):82-9.

The Foundational Sciences and Third-Year Clerkships

Elizabeth Werley, MD, FACEP
Associate Residency Program Director
Penn State Hershey

Susan B. Promes, MD, MBA, FACEP
Professor and Chair
Penn State Hershey

Every core rotation in medical school has relevance to the practice of emergency medicine.

Medical school can be viewed as having two distinct periods of learning: the preclinical and clinical years. Depending on the institution, the training in the foundational sciences (preclinical coursework) generally takes up the first 18 months to 2 years of medical school. Clinical rotations make up the latter half of medical school. The way you learn the material, the type of exams you experience and the manner in which you are evaluated differ vastly in these two different stages of your education. Not surprisingly, emergency medicine residency program selection committees evaluate and weigh the various components of your medical school experience differently. Performance on clinical rotations is among the most important aspects of your application.

That being said, a well-rounded candidate is typically the strongest candidate. Every program director would love to have the smartest medical students in their residency program. But the intelligent and well-rounded applicant is a true catch. Extracurricular and scholarly activities in addition to a strong academic track record demonstrate that an applicant has time management and organizational skills, that they are able to accomplish difficult activities, such as working on a research project or being involved in an organization, all while still maintaining appropriate grades. The student who is involved with extracurricular and scholarly activities but does not have the strongest grades may be perceived as not having their priorities appropriately aligned, or not have the ability to balance their activities with their education. Therefore, these activities add to the strength of an application, but the foundation remains your educational performance.

The Foundational Sciences: No Red Flags

An easy way to sum up the first part of medical school, the foundational sciences or preclinical years, is to stress the importance of having no "red flags" on your record. In terms of residency applications, your clerkship and elective grades are far more important than your basic science grades. You want to have a *minimum* goal of passing all of your basic science classes. After you become a doctor no one ever asks what grade you earned in pathophysiology or pharmacology. The goal is to pass your classes. Of course, if your school offers honors or is on the letter grade system, an "A" will never hurt you.

Any red flags, such as a failed course, will need to be explained in your residency application. If you have a legitimate reason for poor performance, such as a personal/family emergency, and it is an isolated incident, you might be surprised to find that many residency programs are very forgiving. However, when you start to accumulate more than one red flag, programs start to question if there is a pattern, and you will likely struggle when it comes to getting a residency in emergency medicine.

However, don't assume you can get away with achieving the bare-bones minimum, either. Consider every grade of honors or its institutional equivalent as a bonus, and these bonuses are cumulative. Receiving a grade of honors also increases the likelihood of being nominated for Alpha Omega Alpha (AOA) or other regional and national academic awards. Membership in organizations such AOA stands out on applications. Unless your school is strictly pass/fail on every class and/or rotation, eventually you get ranked and sorted amongst your peers. When your medical school prepares your Medical Student Performance Evaluation (MSPE) or dean's letter as part of the residency application process, you will likely be numerically ranked or placed in a performance category compared to your peers. Some schools do not use strict numerical rankings, but may give ranks by fractions of your class, whether it be by thirds, quarters, quartiles, etc.; other schools may make more descriptive distinctions as to your candidacy, such as "outstanding" versus "excellent" versus "good." The better your performance in the pre-clinical years, the higher up you go in the various ranking systems.

So how does one do well in the basic sciences in medical school? The simple answer is to study. Since the content of the foundational sciences may be presented in a different format than you are used to, or you may have never covered certain topics in your undergraduate career, you may be forced to alter your prior study habits. Medicine builds on itself, so cramming before each test will likely be to your detriment as you build your knowledge base. Use a variety of study techniques. If you used to read alone, try studying in groups. If you survived on pulling all-nighters and cramming the day before an exam, trying setting aside a minimum amount of time to read each day. If you used to study quietly in the library, but that doesn't seem to work much anymore, go outside or try a coffee shop. If you used to prefer a noisy background, but now find it too distracting, invest in earplugs, noise-cancelling headphones, or a device that produces white noise in the background.

With the current and evolving technology, today's learners are accustomed to a fast-paced world where a wealth of information is literally at their fingertips. These same learners absorb little bits of data better, compared to previous generations who may have preferred to read an entire textbook chapter in one sitting. If you take a train or carpool, use that time to review material on an app or program. If you do set aside large chunks of time to study in a more traditional fashion, build breaks into your schedule. Be sure to build small rewards into your schedule as well. If you feel like you accomplished your studying goals for the day, and you ended earlier than the time you allotted, take that extra time for yourself. Have dinner with your friends, see the movie you've been waiting for, catch up on your favorite show or current book. Don't be afraid to rearrange your study schedule from time to time. If you don't seem to be grasping a concept, instead of getting frustrated and angry or disappointed with yourself, push the "reset" button. It's amazing what a quick run, a short coffee break, or just a 5-minute phone conversation can do to refresh you and clear your mind.

One other important aspect to studying the basic sciences, or any course of study, is to make sure you ask for help, and do it early, if you find yourself struggling. There is a reason more institutions are incorporating problem-based learning and small group discussions into the education process. Not only does this generation of learners prefer their information in short topics, but group-based learning and a team approach is critical. Use this to your advantage. If you cannot sufficiently grasp a concept, ask someone else for assistance, because s/he might be able to walk you through the steps or present the material in a different light. If you do not want to ask a classmate, you can always ask a more senior student in your school, or even better, a helpful resident or faculty member, because they understand the practical application of the knowledge you're trying to learn. When you change your perspective, it can change your perception and ultimate retention of a topic.

Third-Year Clerkships: The Time to Shine

Next come your clinical rotations. This is an important time to shine for students interested in emergency medicine, given our specialty is all about the clinical practice of medicine. Every school will have a slightly varied structure of required clerkships, but most commonly, the core rotations are internal medicine, surgery, OB/gyn, and pediatrics. Note that not every medical school has a required EM clerkship. You want to do as well as possible on these rotations. Make sure you understand what elements of your performance are used to decide your grade. Who actually has input into your grade? How much does the end of rotation exam (if one is given) count toward your grade? Get to know your patients well. Learn as much as you can from every patient you see. Find a pearl to remember on a patient from rounds, even if it's not a patient you are primarily following. Play an active role in rounds. Ask thoughtful questions. Try to anticipate the needs of your team. Be a team player. Of note, being nice and having pleasant, professional interactions with your patients is important. However, if those are the only comments about you from your supervising residents and faculty, that says something. If you are pleasant, hard-working, and knowledgeable, your evaluations will say such, which will have a much stronger impact on your final grade for that clerkship and on your residency application.

You may not enjoy all of your required rotations, but since emergency medicine incorporates the knowledge and skills from all the various areas of medicine, every rotation is relevant to the daily practice of this specialty. One suggestion to make rotations more enticing is to find how each clinical rotation relates to emergency medicine. If you are on your surgery rotation, practice your wound care skills. If you are on OB/gyn, try to get involved in or at least observe a complicated delivery. On internal medicine, when you see a new patient, try to determine what your treatment plan would have been had the patient presented to you in the ED. On pediatrics, it can be heartbreaking to care for a sick or terminally ill child, but it's an inevitable part of our field, so the earlier you expose yourself to it, the better. These are just a few examples. The residents and faculty supervising you will take note of your enthusiasm and, assuming your fund of knowledge is at least reasonable, your clerkship evaluations will likely reflect this. One of the greatest honors you could receive at the end of a rotation is for someone to try to recruit you to his/her specialty because of your performance on the clerkship.

Although it is somewhat of a cliché, there is a lot of truth about the importance of "being a team player," especially on your clerkship rotations. Your "team" is bigger than you may think. It extends well beyond the usual players of senior students, residents, or faculty. Don't forget to involve those other personnel taking care of the patient along with you — nurses, techs and aides, respiratory therapists, social work, etc. If you are friendly with them and treat them with respect, you would be surprised how much it will be to your advantage. Nurses might save procedures for you. They might even throw good cases your way, or even clinical suggestions that make you look like a rock star on rounds. You can use this opportunity to get good at IV access, which is a skill critical to emergency medicine. A skilled tech might teach you how to do an ECG or hook someone up to the telemetry monitor. Learning how ECG leads are placed on a patient will aide in your basic understanding and interpretation of the actual electrocardiogram. Techs and aides might help you with splinting or dressing changes on wounds. Respiratory therapists might be the first ones to actually help you interpret and understand a blood gas in a real clinical setting, compared to some acid/base talk you sat through in medical school. Social work might help clue you in on details regarding your patient's care. Talk with them to see if there are any roadblocks in your patient's care or ultimate disposition. It may be something as simple as ambulation, so try to walk your patient. Those who cannot walk may need long-term rehab or a nursing home, or if their oxygen saturation drops, they may need further work-up or supplemental oxygen at home. These things take time to arrange, but if you bring it to the attention of your team, not only have you helped your patient, but you look like a student who can see the "big picture."

These same people can help you be properly prepared for rounds. One good tip is to go in extra early. You need to examine the patient and review any notes from earlier in the day or the day prior. You also need to review any laboratory or imaging results, as well as the patient's vital signs. Ask the nurses about any major events overnight, or if they learned anything in sign-out from their overnight colleagues; this small action might draw your attention to something relevant that others may have missed or were unaware of. If a patient just recently developed a fever, the on-call resident might not know yet. A good nurse probably already drew blood cultures and will tell you this, so when it comes time to round, suggest ordering blood cultures and hanging antibiotics, and you get credit for the "good catch." Don't forget to pay back these favors from the staff, either. If you have important tests that need to be urgently resulted, tell the nurses you'll run them to the lab so they don't have to. Staying a little late to help wrap up a care plan for the day also does not go unnoticed. Quid pro quo is an important lesson not just for medicine, but for life.

Come in early and pre-round on your patients. You will then have your workday, when the care team rounds on patients. There will be studies to follow up. Patients will need re-assessment, especially after any interventions. New patients may require admission to your service. You may stay late to help wrap things up for the day. You might be thinking to yourself, when will there be time to study? The answer to that question might be more of a relief than an actual concern.

An easy way to study when on your clinical clerkships is to read a little bit each day. Take one aspect of your patient's care and read 15-30 minutes on it each night. One night you might want to read on the appropriate work-up needed to make the diagnosis. Another night you can focus on the differential diagnosis or mimics of the condition. Another night could be treatment options. If you are ambitious and productive, or if you've been following the same patient for several days, start reading a little bit on other interesting patients on your team. Not only are you learning, but also you'll be able to participate on rounds even more, and really stand out. If you're on a specialty service with a narrower focus, such as gastroenterology, and not a general medicine rotation, there are likely recommended readings given during the orientation for your internal medicine clerkship. Make sure to read these along the way, to ensure you are learning the topics you need to know. If this seems overwhelming, find topics that relate to your patient's past medical history, or someone else you know, whether that is a friend or family member. If a medical condition has a personal relation, you are more likely to remember it. Another helpful tip is always have something to read; there is frequently "down-time" on a rotation. Use that time to build relationships and study. Make sure you get plenty of rest so you are at your best the next day.

If there is a skill involved with an aspect of your rotation, practice it for a few minutes each night. If you are on your surgery rotation, be sure to take home some suture material each night, and practice tying your knots, or borrow a suture kit and practice suturing on inanimate objects, such as bananas, hot dogs, or foam. If you're on internal medicine, review electrocardiogram interpretation. On pediatrics, review basic doses of weight-based medications or IV fluids that you will use routinely, or tricks for remembering appropriate vital signs by age. On OB/gyn, review monitor strips, the stages of delivery, or maneuvers that can be done in a difficult delivery. You can easily get bored if you're only reading at night, for long periods of time. If you interrupt reading with skills practice, not only do you get a break, but also you reinforce topics you've read about. The added benefit is that practical application of your newfound knowledge is more likely to reinforce the material than just reading.

You cannot and should not read, review, and practice around the clock. Just like studying with your foundational sciences, you need to take breaks for down-time. You need to take care of yourself. Even if it's as simple as working out, going for a coffee break, or watching your favorite show, be sure to take time to decompress. It is during this time in your training when you will really develop and practice your time management skills. This pertains to your time away from the hospital as well as the actual clinical setting. Good sleep hygiene is a must to survive and thrive in medicine.

It is good to keep in mind that the residents on service with you are likely contributing to your evaluation and are definitely contributing to your education. If they suggest a coffee break or invite you to the cafeteria for lunch, go with them. It shows you are a team player who can interact appropriately in a social setting. It shows you are human. If you get along with the residents on your service, and you've demonstrated your fund of knowledge on rounds, your residents are more likely to involve you in more interesting cases or procedures. This is where your foundational sciences vary greatly with your clinical clerkships. The social dynamics involved in the actual practice of medicine go far beyond book knowledge.

The Practice of Emergency Medicine

How does all of this relate to emergency medicine? The short answer is that everything is relevant. You will need a strong knowledge base, since emergency physicians need to be prepared for anything that can come through the door. There is little predictability as to the timing or acuity of patient care in the ED, so your skills at multi-tasking and time management are critical. Even the social aspects of medicine that you discovered on your clerkships apply to the variety of social dynamics you may encounter in the ED. In addition to your medical knowledge, there is a wide array of skills you are responsible for as an emergency physician. Summed up, if there is one specialty that potentially applies all of the knowledge you obtained during your foundational sciences and your clinical clerkships, it is emergency medicine.

Extracurricular Activities

Jill Corbo, MD, RDMS
Assoc. Professor
Jacobi Medical Center Albert Einstein College of Medicine

Tina Sundaram, MD
Emergency Medicine Resident
Jacobi/Montefiore Emergency
Medicine Residency Program

David Reid, DO
Emergency Medicine Resident
UT Southwestern/Parkland
Memorial Hospital

One of the most important things you can do is to get involved in activities outside your academic endeavors.

Emergency medicine is one of the fastest growing and most competitive specialties, and residency programs consider not only students' scores, but also their many extracurricular activities. These qualities and experiences can help differentiate you from your peers amid the intense competition for residency positions. This is not, however, a competition for the most bullet points on a resume. Remember that anything you list as a work experience, special interest, or hobby is fair game in an interview, so be prepared to have a good story and worthwhile explanation for its relevance on your application. Quality over quantity is most important when it comes to extracurricular activity, and it can be particularly important for EM applicants. A retrospective study conducted by UC San Diego's Department of Emergency Medicine assessed potential predictors of future success in EM residents and found that "distinctive factors" such as "being involved in national student organizations" correlated well with overall success in EM training.[1] EM programs are looking for "distinctive" candidates, so make sure your application shows how well-rounded you are.

Medical students have tons of opportunities to participate in EM-specific or general medical organizations and interest groups. Start looking for projects and groups that interest you early in your medical school years, but remember that these things often take a lot of time, and while having extracurricular activities on your application is important, it should not be at the expense of your grades. When picking extracurricular activities, it is important to first be clear how much time and involvement is necessary and determine if that fits in with your academic and clinical responsibilities.

Participation in activities and special projects will show your engagement and dedication, but if possible, investigate different leadership opportunities both on and off campus. A leadership position within an organization showcases your ability to simultaneously handle multiple responsibilities, and it can show that you are not only an excellent student, but an enthusiastic future leader for the EM specialty. EM physicians have to be leaders every day, so it is important to take every opportunity to develop this skill early in your career.

On-Campus Opportunities

First and foremost, you should join your medical school's Emergency Medicine Interest Group (EMIG) – aka the "ER Club" – and get involved with all of its various activities. EMIGs help you gain exposure to the field prior to residency and provide a forum for student, resident, and faculty interaction. There will likely be opportunities to learn more about the specialty, participate in skills labs (e.g. suturing and airway technique), shadow faculty physicians, participate in research projects, and attend fun social events. Networking with residents and faculty is a huge benefit of EMIG participation, so take advantage!

EMIG leadership is a great way for you to show you are participating at the next level. There are often several different types of EMIG officer positions for you to shoot for, each with their own unique niche. EMIG leadership is also a fantastic way to coordinate with groups from other medical schools to build regional collegiality and bring new opportunities to students that may not have been made available without inter-institutional cooperation. EMIG leaders across the country have been successful in hosting regional advising events and residency fairs, or even technical skills labs with activities such as ultrasound instruction or simulation competition. There is so much potential when individual leaders can find ways to combine resources and work together.

If your school does not have an EMIG, start one! Talk to your school's Student Affairs representatives and find out how to create a campus organization. Look for potential faculty advisers and sponsors, such as a clerkship director or EM lecturer.

Finally, playing a role in your school's Student Government Association (SGA) is another great way to work face-to-face with your peers on projects and programs that benefit your classmates. A SGA position looks great on your resume, just like an EMIG leadership position, and it can give you the opportunity to learn how professional and non-profit organizations are managed. This can be an important experience for future leadership roles.

Off-Campus Opportunities

Those who venture a little farther from their medical school grounds will find that an abundance of diverse leadership opportunities exist for students outside of the campus setting. Much like those on campus, these positions can be categorized into EM-focused – such as EMRA's Medical Student Council (MSC) – or more general opportunities through organizations like the American Medical Association (AMA) or the American Medical Student Association (AMSA). These professional societies commonly focus on big-picture issues that affect large portions of their members. Work within these groups typically involves extensive collaboration with representatives from across the country, and progress on certain issues can be slow – but also very rewarding. These positions often require a great deal of extracurricular responsibility, including regular conference calls and significant travel time. So plan accordingly by asking up front what to expect should you be chosen for a position, and make sure you will have the time and ability to be successful.

EMRA is one of the premier organizations offering medical students opportunities to serve as national leaders and committee members in EM. EMRA has a very close relationship with the American College of Emergency Physicians (ACEP), and students can get co-membership in these organizations. There are many additional opportunities, though, and you are encouraged to look around, and find your niche! Following are some great EM-specific and other more general medical organizations that have medical student opportunities:

- American Academy of Emergency Medicine (aaem.org)
- American College of Emergency Physicians (acep.org)
- American College of Osteopathic Emergency Physicians (acoep.org)
- American Medical Association (ama-assn.org)
- American Medical Student Association (amsa.org)
- American Osteopathic Association (osteopathic.org)
- Emergency Medicine Residents' Association (emra.org)
- Society for Academic Emergency Medicine (saem.org)

Other "Extracurricular" Activities

SERVICE AT A FREE CLINIC

Volunteering in a free clinic is another outstanding and well-respected extracurricular activity. Free clinics can help you gain experience working with patients and reinforce what you learn in the classroom. Clinic responsibilities can vary widely, from administrative tasks, to coordinating lab tests, to taking part in the patient care with physician oversight.

RESEARCH

Performing research during medical school is a valuable experience and learning opportunity. The summer between the first and second years is one time to explore any research possibilities. One can get involved in ongoing research projects or cultivate your own ideas. The best source of opportunities for ongoing research is the EM faculty. If you are more ambitious and want to start your own research idea, explore the local and national organizations for grants and mentors that may be available. ACEP state chapters often have research grants available for motivated students and residents (www.acep.org/chapters).

Extracurricular activities can help to differentiate you from your peers amid the intense competition for residency positions. As an EM leader you will learn about all aspects of the specialty, as well as how to manage expectations, relationships, and problems that you would have never otherwise encountered during medical school. Leadership opportunities for students in EM are so much more diverse than the traditional designations of president, vice president, treasurer, etc. Be honest with yourself in what you are most passionate about in medicine. Let that drive your search for a leadership role, whether it's at the EMIG, state chapter, or national organization level. If that is to be in a president or chair's post, then go for it! Make sure you know what responsibilities you are accepting, and remember that working for your peers will not only benefit them, but you as well. Always remember that academic and clinical duties should not be compromised by these outside responsibilities. Holding a leadership opportunity will give you the chance to network with students from around the country as well as the current leaders in EM. Leadership is a trait that is developed and honed over time. It is also a fantastic way to meet mentors, colleagues, and friends that you will collaborate with for the rest of your career.

REFERENCES

1. Hayden SR, Hayden M, Gamst A. "What characteristics of applicants to emergency medicine residency programs predict future success as an emergency medicine resident?" *Acad Emerg Med.* 2005 Mar;12(3):206-10

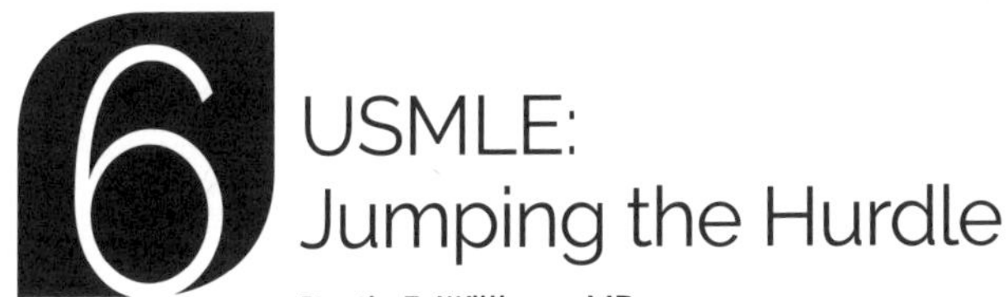

USMLE: Jumping the Hurdle

Dustin B. Williams, MD
Assistant Residency Director
UT Southwestern/Parkland Memorial Hospital

The USMLE (U.S. Medical Licensing Examination) and COMLEX (Comprehensive Osteopathic Medical Licensing Examination) can be points of trepidation for many students applying for an emergency medicine residency program. Medical students are all too familiar with standardized testing. Like an Olympic athlete preparing for competition, long hours will have been spent preparing for these exams. Among the all-time greatest athletes in the women's heptathlon, Jackie Joyner-Kersee garnered multiple gold medals – attributing her success to dedication, determination, and desire. The same can be said for preparing for the boards. Taking the USMLE is just another hurdle in the process of becoming a board-certified emergency physician. The results of your board testing can significantly impact your ability to gain entry into the program of your choice, so knowing what program directors are looking for, particularly in the area of test scores, will be valuable to overcoming hurdles and to realistically assessing your candidacy for the program you desire.

> ***Because board scores are standardized, they are the only objective part of a student's application.***

A Program Director's Perspective

Program directors (PDs) take many attributes into consideration when examining candidates. While a student's letters of recommendation and dean's letter are important factors in selecting applicants to interview, a recent survey of emergency medicine program directors indicated the USMLE Step 1 and COMLEX Level 1 scores were the most important factor.[2] Many programs, for example, use the USMLE Step 1 as a screening tool when deciding upon applicants to interview. Those with scores below a certain threshold are, often times, automatically disqualified from further consideration. According to a 2014 survey of emergency medicine program directors, 69 percent indicated they wanted program candidates to have a target score on USMLE Step 1 or COMLEX Level 1, when deciding which applicants to interview.[2] Those target scores will vary by program, so in order to maximize your chances for an interview, it is important to do your best on these exams while taking into consideration the other key components cited by PDs, such as letters of recommendation, clerkship scores, grades, extracurricular activities and sometimes personal statements.[5]

Trends in USMLE

Several trends are apparent in USMLE Step 1 and 2 scores for emergency medicine program applicants. Since 2009, the average USMLE Step 1 scores for U.S. seniors who successfully matched in emergency medicine have steadily increased from an average of 222 to an average of 230 in 2014. Step 2 scores have shown similar trends, increasing from 230 in 2009 to 243 in 2014.[3] These numbers illustrate a trend in higher scoring among those matching in emergency medicine programs and underscore the competitive nature of today's EM residency programs.

> ***The numbers illustrate a trend in higher scoring among those matching in emergency medicine programs.***

What Are Your Options?

Because many emergency medicine program directors use board scores as a screening tool for selecting applicants to interview, some students are left questioning the definition of a good score. In a 2013 survey of program directors, when asked what score they felt represented one that would likely be granted an interview, the average "good" score reported was 240, with a range of 230-250.[2] Table 1 shows mean scores of matched and unmatched EM applicants in 2014.

TABLE 1. HOW DID EM CANDIDATES SCORE?

Mean USMLE Step 1 score
Matched U.S. Seniors: 230; Unmatched: 215
Matched Independent Applicants: 226; Unmatched: 217
Mean USMLE Step 2 score
Matched U.S. Seniors: 243; Unmatched: 225
Matched Independent Applicants: 237; Unmatched: 225

Source: "Charting Outcomes in the Match, 2014," NRMP

Given the importance of these scores in identifying successful matches, your score on USMLE Step 1 can impact the timing in which you take Step 2. Generally, program directors will send interview invitations when applicants present with an acceptable Step 1 score in conjunction with a solid application, even without a reported Step 2 score. But if your Step 1 score is less desirable than you hoped, it may be wise to take Step 2 CK earlier in order to bolster your application. In a recent survey of program directors, 94 percent reported they strongly consider Step 2 CK when selecting interview candidates.[2] This statistic provides strong motivation to take USMLE Step 2 by August 31 in order to have your scores reported by October 1. Regarding Step 2 CS, program directors place less emphasis on this exam when determining interview invitations, but you must pass it in order to successfully match.

Deciding on when to take the USMLE Step 2 can be anxiety-provoking for the residency applicant. If an applicant's Step 1 score is less desirable than hoped for, it may be wise to take Step 2 CK earlier in order to bolster the application. Recently, program directors have begun placing more emphasis on Step 2 scores because the content of Step 2 tends to be more clinically relevant. In a recent survey of program directors, 94 percent reported they strongly consider Step 2 CK when selecting interview candidates.[2] This encourages many applicants to take USMLE Step 2 by August 31 in order to have scores reported by October 1. While having a stellar USMLE Step 2 score can make up for a suboptimal Step 1 score, having a poor Step 2 score can overshadow a solid Step 1 performance. If you fall below the mean or are unhappy with you score, and you are confident your score can be improved, then it is advisable to take Step 2 early in order to improve your application. Many programs prefer to see Step 2 scores prior to offering interview invitations; however, very few programs actually require it. Regarding Step 2 CS, program directors place less emphasis on this exam when determining interview invitations, but a student does need to ensure it is passed in order to successfully match as a failure on this exam can be a major red flag to program directors.

Word of caution. Don't get overly panicked if your scores aren't as high as you hoped. Students with scores in the 200-230 range can and do successfully match each year. If you don't think your score is as competitive as the average applicant's, build up other areas of your application and stand out in other ways. It is essential to speak with your adviser or clerkship director early if you think your board score may hinder your ability to match. This will allow you to develop an early plan for successfully applying and matching.

COMLEX and ACGME: Not Just Alphabet Soup

Students in allopathic medical schools are required to take the USMLE, while students in osteopathic programs take the COMLEX. Some osteopathic medical school graduates may wish to pursue an allopathic residency upon completion of medical school. This brings into question whether they should take the USMLE in order to successfully match. In a word, yes.

Because board scores are standardized, they are the only universal objective assessment as part of a student's application. However, when two different boards are involved — allopathic vs. osteopathic — comparing the scores can be difficult. Recent research has shown that osteopathic students who report USMLE scores are 1.5 times more likely to successfully match into an ACGME program. Further, 77 percent of program directors in the same survey said it was at least somewhat important for osteopathic students pursuing allopathic residency to report a USMLE score.[4] Therefore, if you're an osteopathic student interested in pursuing an allopathic residency, your best bet is to take the USMLE in addition to the COMLEX, in order to have the greatest likelihood of matching.

REFERENCES

1. http://womenshistory.about.com/od/quotes/a/joyner_kersee.htm
2. Results of the 2014 NRMP Program Directory Survey. June 2014. NRMP. available at www.nrmp.org
3. Liang, M. Charting outcomes in the Match. 5th Edition. August 2014. available at www.nrmp.org
4. Weizberg, M. Should Osteopathic Students applying to Allopathic Emergency Medicine Programs Take the USMLE Exam? *West J Emerg Med.* 2013;XV(1)
5. CORD. http://www.cordem.org/files/DOCUMENTLIBRARY/2015%20AA/PLD%20Handouts/Making_an_Effective_Rank_List.pdf

For more information, please see the Medical Student Survival Guide *online at emra.org.*

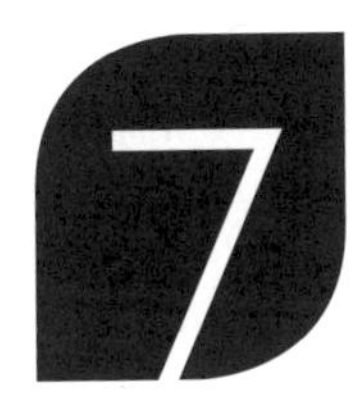

Fourth Year and Emergency Medicine Rotations

Jeremy Sperling, MD, FACEP
Chairman, Department of Emergency Medicine
Jacobi Medical Center and North Central Bronx Hospital

Jonathan St. George, MD
Faculty Coordinator, Subinternship in Emergency Medicine
New York Presbyterian Hospital/Weill Cornell Medical Center

Scheduling Rotations and Obtaining Letters of Recommendation/SLOEs

Now that you have decided emergency medicine is the right specialty for you, it's time to schedule your EM rotations, which give you the opportunity to be true providers, not merely observers of care. This supervised opportunity makes every EM rotation valuable. The hands-on clinical experience lets you demonstrate how you will perform as a resident, and your evaluations from these rotations carry a lot of weight with EM program directors and could greatly influence your match.

Make sure your fourth year is about obtaining a fantastic educational and clinical experience.

It's very important when making rotation decisions to be aware of the timeline and logistics of the residency application process and to make sure your rotation choices will support your goal of matching in emergency medicine. Although this chapter deals with the logistics of setting up your fourth-year rotations and obtaining letters of recommendation, it is necessary to keep things in perspective. First and foremost make sure your fourth year is about obtaining a fantastic educational and clinical experience. Although this can be a stressful time, have fun and enjoy your fourth year, which has the potential to be the best year of medical school.

Emergency medicine candidates should aim for two EM rotations. Typically one of these is at your home institution, and the other is an "away rotation" at another clinical site that has an EM residency program. Ideally, the "away" rotation is at a program you are highly considering for residency. If your school does not have an EM residency program, then you may need to do two away rotations. Doing more than two months of EM is not necessary, but in certain circumstances may be considered. Even if you are certain EM is the right choice for you, your fourth year of medical school remains a unique opportunity to experience the breadth of medicine. Instead of overdoing it on EM rotations, get clinical experience that is relevant to the practice of EM. Examples might include pediatrics, critical care, anesthesia, orthopedics, toxicology, and radiology.

Having your application ready to be released on the first day the applications are accepted is optimal. If you can get at least one EM letter of recommendation in your application when the system launches, it can help you get interviews. In order to accomplish this, you will have to complete an EM rotation at least a couple of weeks before the acceptance period begins. A September "away" rotation is fairly standard, but the downside can be that your letter of recommendation for this rotation might not make it into your application until mid-October! It may seem early, but you should consider July and August as prime months for EM rotations.

Research EM rotation options early. You are not only researching potential elective months, but also where you might want to match for your residency. Important considerations when choosing a rotation and residency program include your career goals (e.g., academics, community, subspecialty training) and geography (i.e., where you want to live). Also consider the experience previous students have had at that clinical site. Talk to prior participants to find out: Do students have the opportunity to be primary care providers to patients? Is there a lot of bedside teaching? Is there an organized didactic or simulation curriculum? Have former students received a lot of mentorship from the faculty? Does the program appear to recruit a lot of their residents from students who rotated there?

When choosing electives, consider rotations whose formats and styles complement each other. As an example, your two clinical rotations may combine a highly academic tertiary care program and a large public hospital setting; a 4-year and a 3-year residency program; or a community-based program and an academic program. Choosing rotations that differ in fundamental ways will provide you with firsthand insights into the nature of different residency programs. This could later help you make an educated decision about the types of programs where you will want to apply and eventually match. On the other hand, if you are already very confident about the type of program you want, then concentrate on programs with that format. For example, if you know you want a 4-year, highly academic residency program, then it might make more sense to do all of your rotations at clinical sites with this format.

Although EM rotations at clinical sites that do not have an EM residency program can be highly educational, they are not as helpful when it comes to making connections and improving your chances of matching in a residency program. An EM away rotation at a residency program is a networking opportunity that you should take full advantage of. It is an incredibly common occurrence for students to match at programs where they rotated during their fourth year.

It is smart to schedule your "home" clerkship as your first EM rotation. Utilize your home rotation to learn the basics of EM, to make sure EM is the right specialty for you, and to obtain a SLOE. Complete this first rotation as soon as possible, definitely by the end of August at the latest. Remember, if your school doesn't have a home program, you should be ready to schedule two rotations at other institutions.

Scheduling Your "Away" EM Rotation

As stated, the goal for the "away" rotation beyond learning EM is to evaluate if that residency program would be a good fit for you, and vice versa. Additionally, it is an opportunity to get a strong SLOE letter. Make sure this away rotation is somewhere you would want to live. Doing an away elective can be expensive; however, after the expense of medical school, this 1-month investment, if it helps you match in your "dream" program, could be well worth it. There are ways to find affordable arrangements. The AAMC Visiting Student Applications Service (VSAS) page has a link to one potential resource called rotating room: http://rotatingroom.com.

There are a few reasons to consider extra EM rotations. If you are concerned about the competitiveness of your EM application, an extra rotation will allow another residency program to get to know you and understand how interested you are in their program. Geography might be a factor as well. If you have to match in a specific city or you want to match in a very competitive region of the country, you might want to do multiple EM rotations to increase your chances. Finally, you may just want an extra rotation to obtain exposure to different types of programs. Word of caution: Be sure to get a SLOE for each EM rotation to avoid raising any questions during your interviews. Emergency medicine is a tightly connected community, so deciding to not ask for a SLOE because you're not sure it will be a glowing recommendation won't stop program directors from calling your rotation sites to see how you performed. If you're concerned about a bad recommendation, discuss it with the EM clerkship director.

Scheduling Other Types of EM Rotations

There are other ways to gain ED exposure besides the traditional ED rotation, such as ultrasound, toxicology, or EMS. These are outstanding educational experiences, but know that a letter from one of these may not be as valuable or as relevant to your application, and the structure and value may vary greatly from place to place.

Visiting Student Application Services (VSAS)

The Visiting Student Application Services of the Association of American Medical Colleges is a service that allows medical students to complete an online application and to apply for senior electives at other United States medical schools. The website (https://services.aamc.org/20/vsas) lists all the participating medical schools, their individual requirements, elective dates, and procedures and dates for applying to each institution. Carefully review this information and be ready to send in your full applications at the earliest dates possible. Have in mind back-up plans in case you do not get your first choice of "away" rotations.

Fourth Year Medical School Scheduling Tips

If you have a mandatory rotation in a field other than emergency medicine (e.g., internal medicine, pediatrics) or another mandatory rotation, avoid scheduling these other requirements in the July through September blocks when you must be concentrating on EM rotations. Also, be strategic about what you schedule during the interview season, which may go from mid-November through January. Try to ensure your rotations offer you some schedule flexibility so you can attend interviews.

> *The SLOE is designed to be a "global" evaluation.*

Beyond your EM clerkships, make sure you will complete all of your medical school graduation requirements with cushion built into your system, to guarantee you will be able to graduate on time. Don't risk matching in the residency program and field of your dreams and then not graduating on time because you missed a requirement.

Standard Letter of Evaluation (SLOE)

Emergency medicine clerkship directors (CDs) will expect you to ask them for a Standard Letter of Evaluation at the completion of your EM rotation. Many CDs will mention how to get a SLOE during the clerkship orientation. If they don't comment on the process during orientation, ask them early in the rotation how obtaining a SLOE works in their department.

A SLOE is different than other letters for your application. The SLOE is intended to be a letter of evaluation, not necessarily a letter of recommendation. The SLOE is designed to be a "global" evaluation of how you did on your EM rotation, and it is designed to compare you against your colleagues in terms of your clinical skills as well your potential as an emergency medicine resident. The form asks letter writers to compare you against your colleagues in areas such as commitment to EM, work ethic, ability to work as a team, communication skills, and amount of guidance you would require. The form is online (www.cordem.org/i4a/pages/index.cfm?pageid=3743); you should review it prior to starting your EM clerkships.

The form is intended for emergency medicine faculty. Most programs utilize it as a composite evaluation that incorporates feedback from all faculty members you worked with clinically, as well as input from residents or other members of the ED team with whom you may have worked. Additionally, it may include performance on any presentations you gave, simulations and procedures labs you participated in, and final exams (oral and written). A composite SLOE is usually signed by the program director, assistant program directors, and/or the clerkship directors. In some institutions, the whole educational leadership team will sign the letter; in other programs one representative signs the letter on behalf of the program or clerkship.

Individual Faculty Letters of Recommendation

The SLOE can be utilized by an individual faculty member, writing a single letter of recommendation. When reviewing applications, most program directors find a composite EM letter to carry a lot more weight than individual letters of recommendation. Typically, this is because a composite letter or SLOE is a "global" evaluation of a candidate's performance in comparison to others on the rotation, as described above. By contrast, an individual faculty member who might only have spent a few shifts with an applicant is basing his/her assessment on a much more limited amount of information. On the other hand, a letter from an EM faculty member whom you have spent considerable time with, who can therefore write a strong and personal letter with a lot of insight into your character and clinical skills, could still be valuable. A considerable amount of time is not a few shifts, but rather time together working on a research project, a global health experience, or a boutique clinical rotation. Impersonal individual letters from a chairman, PD, or nationally known EM physician will not be particularly useful if they are vague or weak and will not add anything to a department's composite SLOE letter. On the contrary, it could hurt an application if the applicant could have obtained a particularly strong and personal letter from someone else, even if that person is outside of EM.

Number of Letters of Recommendation/SLOEs

Two SLOEs, one from a home institution and one from an away rotation are ideal. If you have a third SLOE, include it, but it is certainly not required. A major reason for completing the two main EM rotations early is so the two letters can be in your file when Electronic Residency Application Service (ERAS) application opens to residency program directors. Most applicants submit 3-4 letters of recommendation; a third or fourth letter is typically from a non-EM faculty member. Ideally this is someone who can write a personal and insightful letter about you and your potential.

How to Succeed on an EM Rotation

This is arguably the most closely scrutinized section, routinely pored over by students in the hopes of finding a prescription for doing well on their EM rotation(s). While there is no magic formula for doing well, Malcolm Gladwell tells us, "Success is not a random act. It arises out of a predictable and powerful set of circumstances and opportunities."[1] It's helpful to remember that your arrival here is not random. You're here because you have shown at this point in your education that you're ready to be here. Take comfort in this fact, commit yourself wholeheartedly to the opportunity, and like so many before you, chances are you will do well.

Those unfamiliar with the emergency department environment may at first see only chaos, but look closer and you will discern a finely tuned and expertly choreographed dance beneath the surface. Here we will break down the basic steps of that dance for you, and in no time you will be functioning as a valued team member during your clerkship. It's important to start out on the right foot – by paying attention to even the most basic details.

Attending physicians are likely to overlook a simple gap in knowledge as something that time and training will correct, but (rightly or wrongly) behaviors and codes of conduct seen as basic or essential to the community you are entering are going to be viewed as a reflection of your character as well as your innate ability to grasp the culture of the department. Missteps in these areas are much more likely to leave a lasting bad impression. The following advice is constructed loosely as a hierarchy of skills for success, with the most fundamental advice first, then working our way up to higher-order performance skills on your EM rotation.

Dress appropriately. There is usually a local ED culture of attire, which might make wearing clean scrubs and/or short white coat acceptable. If you're unsure, dressing conservatively is the wisest option (white coat and business clothing, e.g., for men, shirt, tie, shoes, slacks, and for women, slacks, modest skirts, blouses, closed-toe shoes) until you see what residents and attendings are wearing. There are certain things to avoid even if you see the residents or attendings dressing in this manner. These include sweatshirts, sneakers, unclean or wrinkled white coats or scrubs, political pins, etc. Be clean-shaven and don't show unnecessary skin. Remember this is not only a job, you are also showing up to be someone's doctor. The patients (and likely the attendings and nurses) have never met you; you need to make the right first impression.

Act professionally. Beyond treating the patients and staff extremely well, there are a few things to avoid in the ED setting. Make sure you know the designated places to eat. When you take a food break, make sure you sign out your cases to your senior resident or attendings, and make sure all of your patients have already been presented and their treatment plans are in motion. Do not disappear for long periods of time; always make sure the attending or residents know where you will be in case they need you. Avoid texting, non-job-related Internet surfing, or making personal calls anywhere in sight of patients or in front of your supervising physician. If you have to make a personal call, treat it like a bathroom break and do it outside of the ED. Similarly, avoid personal conversations and joking anywhere within earshot of patients.

Remember, some conduct is mandated by regulatory agencies, and compliance is watched closely by most hospitals. No eating in patient areas is one of these, as is hand hygiene when entering and leaving a patient's room. You do NOT want to be the one who brings down the entire department's hand hygiene score or whose name is on a report to the department about lack of compliance, so follow the rules at all times.

Use good judgment, and never act independently. If a patient appears acutely ill or requires an emergent procedure, tell a senior resident or attending right away (and then return to the bedside). Do not worry that you don't yet have the diagnosis or a full history. Recognizing an acutely ill patient is a core skill in EM, and your timely recognition of a sick patient will be seen as a job well done and a huge help to the team. Additionally, if you do not know something or you don't know the plan, make sure you check in with the attending or senior resident. This is especially true before you start telling a patient a treatment plan or giving patients clinical advice (the patient may end up getting mixed messages).

Be courteous and kind to everyone. First and foremost this means caring about your patients. Be respectful of their concerns and their privacy, find out what motivated them to come in, and what they fear about their visit so you can reassure them. Keep them informed and answer their questions. Make your patients feel more comfortable with simple gestures like bringing them a pillow, a blanket, or food if appropriate. A happy patient who views you as his/her doctor and tells the attending so will carry a lot of weight on your evaluations.

The ED is a unique environment. Unlike your medicine or surgery rotations, where your direct exposure to faculty is often only on rounds, in the OR, or in conference, and your interaction with other support staff may be limited, attendings are physically present at all times in the ED. In addition, you will be working side by side with a complex team of diverse players. Clerks, nurses, physician assistants, techs, consultants, administrators, and many others are always around, and they all have a stake in the department. During your interactions handle any unexpected conflict with professionalism and grace. If a problem escalates, politely disengage and alert your supervising attending. Never assume you know whom you're talking to or who they know, and never make derogatory comments about other health care providers to patients or staff. Remember the old adage, "If you don't have anything nice say, then don't say anything at all."

Be a team player. EM is practiced as a team, and a visible interest in joining that team should be apparent to all who interact with you. This does not mean telling everyone how much you like emergency medicine; rather it should show in how you immerse yourself in the rotation. As a student you may feel peripheral or on the sidelines – especially if your notes are duplicative and you can't put in electronic orders. An excellent student is one who can make himself/herself useful to the team and the patients, and who finds ways to have a positive impact during shifts. Here are some pointers:

An excellent student can make himself/herself useful to the team and the patients.

- Take ownership of any patient you are assigned or you have any responsibility for. Keep them informed about delays, answer their questions, and let them know results. Keep the attending informed when there are any changes in the patients' clinical status (e.g., they become sicker, are in pain, altered mental status). Make sure the attending knows when patients are ready for a disposition (i.e., all of their testing is completed).
- Be helpful to the residents. If a patient needs to be transported or requires bagging, or if someone has to irrigate a wound, offer to pitch in. Others will notice, and you likely will get some teaching or a procedure out of the experience.
- Be aware of what's going on in your area, even if you are not assigned to that particular patient, and ask to help. Running to get an LP kit or a bougie from the airway cart may seem like scut work, but in fact it is valuable and shows you are interested and engaged in the work going on around you.

Focus your knowledge. Our patients present to the ED with undifferentiated problems, so we see an incredibly wide range of medical complaints that overlap with all specialties. From the outside, EM physicians are often seen as "jacks of all trades, masters of none." This leads to the misconception that a broad basic knowledge across specialties is sufficient to do well on an EM rotation, when in fact EM training involves a highly specialized and diligently honed set of skills that have been developed to give our patients the best care possible in the emergency department environment. Before the rotation, start focusing your knowledge and align it with the EM environment so that you can convey your understanding of the concerns and the role of EM physicians in the health care system.

From the undifferentiated complaint, we are experts in the early identification, evaluation, and resuscitation of critically ill patients. It would therefore be helpful to know the initial steps in the resuscitation of an unstable patient based on the most likely diagnosis. Examples include the initial management of STEMI, stroke, pulmonary embolism, GI bleed, or sepsis. An understanding of the types of shock and their management would also be high-value knowledge to have at your command.

We are also skilled in the evaluation of risk in the stable patient based on the clinical context of a chief complaint. Since the majority of the patients you will be seeing will be relatively stable, brush up on your risk evaluation for stable patients. Remember, unlike patients admitted to the floor, your patients don't come to the ED complaining of myocardial infarction; they come in citing chest pain. It will be especially useful to review the approach to the most common chief complaints seen in an ED (e.g., abdominal pain, chest pain, headache) and to know the differential of potentially life-threatening or high morbidity "can't miss" diagnoses. One of the criteria on which you will be evaluated is how well you can formulate these EM focused differentials.

Be curious. Immerse yourself in the experience as a way of showing your engagement, by actively seeking knowledge and asking questions. If you have an interesting case, follow up to learn what the final diagnosis was and what happened; if a good moment arises, share the information with the attending. If an attending asks you to look something up, make sure you do, and let him/her know what you found (either in person, on your next shift, or via a brief email). Always look interested and engaged in learning opportunities. Even if it is the middle of the night or it is a busy shift, if an attending or resident wants to teach, then you should participate.

It's also okay to get personal (within reason). Emergency physicians are a diverse group with a broad range of interests that overlap with their chosen profession. If time and the right context permit, it's OK to get to know your attendings: Get to know their teaching styles, their areas of interest and research, and their personalities on a more personal level.

Understand how you are being evaluated. Your performance will be judged on more than just your knowledge base. The attendings and residents will be watching to see how you conduct yourself personally, how you immerse yourself in all aspects of the rotation, how successfully you integrate yourself into the team, and how you treat patients and staff. They will gauge whether you "get" the core concepts of EM care and whether you are enthusiastic and interested in learning. Beyond the residents and attendings, you should assume a full 360-degree evaluation on EM rotations: Everyone from the clerks and housekeepers to the attendings and chair of the department work together closely. Assume that members of the ED staff may have been working together for decades (because many have been). Finally, treat every patient like a family member.

Be yourself and have fun. The advice in this book is meant to help you, but sometimes the tenor of this checklist of do's and dont's can appear as an ominous mountain of rules looming over your upcoming EM rotation. Is big brother constantly watching and waiting to find a flaw in your performance? Yes and no.

You may believe that once you finish medical school and residency, this constant evaluation process will stop. It doesn't. Most of us accept that EM is a high-stakes profession, that we have an immense responsibility to our patients, and constant oversight and evaluation comes with that responsibility. Yet most of us find a way to incorporate this into our practice and still be our own person. We find great satisfaction in coming to work, taking care of patients, and working alongside our colleagues.

REFERENCES

1. Gladwell, Malcolm. *Outliers: The Story of Success*. 1st ed. New York: Little, Brown and Company, 2008, p155.

For more information, please see the Medical Student Survival Guide *online at emra.org.*

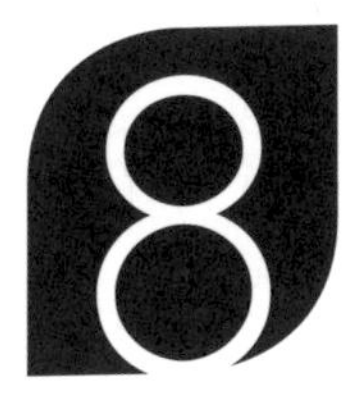

Your Residency Application

Katie Pettit, MD
Assistant Program Director
Indiana University

Carey Chisholm, MD
Program Director Emeritus
Indiana University

> ***Your EM rotation performance is the single most important component of your application.***

Putting together your application for residency is a frequent source of stress for fourth-year medical students. You will likely be asking yourself the following questions: "Am I going to match?" "Should I do an away rotation, and when?" "What goes into my application?" "How many programs should I apply to?" "How many programs should I target for interviews?" "When does my application have to be submitted?" "When should I take Step 2?" This chapter presents a stepwise approach to preparing your application. While every residency program is different, they tend to follow the same timeline and place importance on the same parts of the application.

Assessing Your Strength as a Candidate

"Am I going to match?" Emergency medicine is a competitive specialty. This section explains the components of your application that most EM program directors evaluate in order to decide whether to extend an interview offer.

Your EM rotation(s) performance is the single most important component of your application. Many PDs start their review of your application with this, and the SLOE factors disproportionately into subsequent decisions regarding interview invitations and ranking. This is why every student should get at least two SLOEs from some combination of home and away rotations, keeping in mind that SLOEs generated by EM PDs/faculty carry more credibility. If you desire to do an additional EM rotation that is not at a residency affiliated institution, that is fine, but PDs will put less weight on those SLOEs.

Critical Recommendation #1. Have SLOEs from at least 2 different institutions with EM residencies.

Clinical rotation grades and class ranking also impact your application. PDs tend to place the most emphasis on performance on the internal medicine, surgery, pediatrics, and OB/gyn rotations. These rotations lay an important foundation for future success in emergency medicine, and most PDs desire a strong performance in these core clinical skills. Your class ranking is important but can be more difficult for programs to use as a comparative criterion. In general, the lower the class ranking, the less competitive the applicant. However, if you have performed much better during your MSIII year as compared to your first two years, this is also considered and will work to your advantage. Many medical schools are Pass/Fail only, and this makes it harder for programs to interpret how you performed during your clerkships. There are no distinguishing features between the top performers and those who struggled. This frequently results in the default assumption that you fall in the middle of your class. In these situations, it is critical that your SLOEs reflect your competitive performance.

Next, programs evaluate your USMLE/COMLEX scores. The truth is that these scores are the sole common objective comparative parameter amongst applicants. Filters in the ERAS program permit PDs to set cutoff scores for both Step 1 and Step 2. Many programs desire your Step 2 CK score as well as Step 1. USMLE scores are covered in more depth in Chapter 6, but in general a failure on any Step is bad. It is difficult to match with a failure on USMLE (but not impossible). It is possible to recover from a failed Step 1 score if you do very well on Step 2. A failure on Step 2, especially the CK exam, is almost insurmountable.

Critical Recommendation #2. A poor performance on Step 1 may screen you out of many applicant pools. Address this through a significantly better performance on Step 2 and robust components in other areas of your application. If the Step 1 score is an aberrancy, address this in your personal statement.

So far we have discussed mainly objective data points. These permit PDs to compare applicants (apples to apples) as best as possible. PDs then turn their attention to other components of your application. These include life experiences, extracurricular activities, research experience, and publications. In other words, this is when your CV is analyzed. These experiences and activities will give some applicants the "X" factor, but you have to have made the "cuts" in the objective data in order for the PD to even review these components. Strength in these components often resonates with an individual program's values.

PDs expect an explanation for any blemishes on your record. The least damaging is an isolated clerkship test failure (assuming successful remediation.) The most damaging are in areas of professionalism and conduct. If you have been cited for inability to communicate and interact well on a team, it does not bode well for your likelihood to match. Any legal blemishes (e.g. DUI or arrest) must be explained.

Critical Recommendation #3. Any "blemishes" in your record must be explained in a straightforward fashion. This is best accomplished in the Personal Statement, but may be done in the MSPE.

Finally, program directors expect an understanding of the EM profession and what true practice in EM entails. Applicants frequently talk about the excitement of EM, saving lives, and taking care of the sickest patients and the worst traumas. Although this is an important part of our specialty, non-acute ED visits make up the vast majority of patients. Most patients will be discharged from the ED and will not require any type of procedure. Most programs expect a more in-depth understanding of the practice of EM as opposed to a Personal Statement perseverating on the features that resonate with an adrenaline junkie.

Back to the question, "Will I match?" You need to carefully reflect on your performance in all of the previously discussed areas. If you fall short, you need an honest discussion with your faculty adviser that considers your likelihood of matching. It may be critical to develop a Plan B.

Application Time: Choosing the Type and Number of Programs

This is usually the most difficult part of the application process. During the past 5-10 years, the number of programs the individual applicant applies to has greatly inflated due to the relative ease of applying to additional programs through ERAS, disregard of (or poor) faculty adviser recommendations, and a false belief that this will improve your chances of matching in EM. However, despite the increasing numbers of applications, the likelihood of matching has not changed.[1] In fact, strong applicants accepting more interview spots than necessary is detrimental and unfair to other applicants. Please take this fact into serious consideration when accepting interviews. Your competitiveness, gauged by the information provided in this chapter, serves as a general guide to the number of applications you should submit. Your EM faculty adviser can assist with this process. These are general guidelines for the numbers of programs you should apply to:

Top 10% applicant: Apply to 15-20 programs and interview at 6-10.
Top 25% applicant: Apply to 20-25 programs and interview at 8-12.
Top 50% applicant: Apply to 30 programs and interview at 10-15.
3rd quartile applicant: Apply to 30 - 40 programs and interview at 15-20 (if possible.)
Bottom quartile applicant: Apply to 40 or more programs and interview everywhere you are invited. If you fall into this category, we urge you to have a backup plan as well.

Caveat: *Large numbers of applications do not increase the chances of an invitation to interview for 3rd and 4th quartile applicants. Careful selection, using data from your faculty advisers, allows you to target programs where you have a higher chance of securing an interview. One key question would be "Where have previous grads from our school with similar records successfully matched?"*

In general, programs that are located in geographically less desirable areas or in less ideal climates will have fewer applicants. Less competitive applicants should consider targeting these programs. Keep in mind that just because they are less desirable from a geographical standpoint, it does not mean they are lower quality programs. In some cases, it is quite the opposite. The same thing applies to new programs (those that have only been around 1-2 years,) as they also usually have lower applicant to position ratios.

All of the EM programs in the country have to go through a rigorous accreditation process.

Fortunately (and perhaps confusingly) there is a wide range of EM program training philosophies, patient mixture, and "value added" experiences. There are both 3- and 4-year programs. Some programs are located in an urban environment, while others are rural-based. Identify the environments where you excelled during the academic process and consider seeking similar conditions for your residency. One way to begin evaluating a program is to inquire what recent graduates from the residency program are doing. This will give you a better idea of the opportunities that will be available after graduation. Then ask yourself if that is what you would like to do when you graduate. The good news is that all of the EM programs in the country have to go through a rigorous accreditation process, and you will get solid to excellent training at any of them. Remember that the location and duration of your residency training should be secondary to laying a foundation for a successful 30+ year EM career.

Finally, if you are a Doctor of Osteopathy (DO) or an international medical graduate (IMG), look carefully at the current residents, recent graduates, and faculty at each residency program. While many programs accept both DOs and IMGs, if you do not see anyone like you in the program, you may not have a strong chance of being accepted.

Actual Elements of the ERAS Application

The elements of your ERAS application are listed below. It is imperative that you are honest about your entire application. Do not try to inflate your accomplishments or involvement in activities. EM physicians have a strong "BS meter" and have been trained to sniff this out. Program directors and residents are very adept at determining if you have inflated your accomplishments during the interview process. Misrepresenting information in your CV will ensure you do not match. EM is a tight-knit community, and PDs often discuss applicants with each other.

1. **Demographics.** There is a form in ERAS for all of your personal information.
2. **Medical school transcript.** Find out if you are responsible for loading this into ERAS or if your medical school will do this for you.
3. **USMLE scores.** These are released by the applicant.
4. **Letters of Recommendation.** You can have up to 4 letters. Ideally, at least 2 of these are SLOEs from your EM rotations.
5. **Dean's letter (MSPE).** Medical schools release and upload the dean's letter on the same date for each applicant. This is not a letter of recommendation, but rather a summary of your performance in medical school.
6. **Curriculum Vitae.** This is a list of activities and accomplishments. There is a standardized format in ERAS. Again, be honest about your degree of involvement.
7. **Personal Statement.** This portion of the application usually causes the most stress for applicants. This should be a succinct, one-page document that explains your story. Tell the program director who you are, how you got where you are, and why you are a great EM applicant. You will notice that the personal statement is not listed as one of the more important documents in determining your competitiveness. It is rare that a personal statement will result in an interview offer for someone who would otherwise not be invited. However, a very poorly written personal statement may cause a program to withhold an interview invitation.

Timeline: When Should Everything Be Completed?

Securing an away rotation is the first thing you need to accomplish. Start applying to away rotations during March or April of your third year. You will want to schedule your MSIV year such that you can complete two EM rotations by the end of August. This allows the program to complete your SLOE for inclusion in your file by the beginning of October. If you are a very competitive applicant, you could complete your second EM rotation in September or October. Your second SLOE will not be required for an interview offer if you have performed very well in all other categories.

Begin to assemble your application by June of your MSIV year. Start your personal statement at that time to allow time for revision. Identify who will write your letters of recommendation. To the best extent possible, request these by July. You should have everything ready to upload to ERAS on September 15. This includes your letters of recommendation, personal statement, and CV. If you performed poorly on Step 1, have your Step 2 CK grade into ERAS by mid-October.

The timeline for interview offers depends on the program; it generally begins in October and continues through December as applicants cancel and programs extend offers to those on their wait list. Interviews occur October-January.

Our final piece of advice is to stay in touch with your EM adviser during this entire process. If you receive fewer interview offers than anticipated by an expected time, you need to evaluate why this is the case. Review your application to make sure it is complete. Reconsider your competitiveness as a candidate. Revisit the need for a backup plan. In our experience, 5 or fewer interview offers by December 1 places you at higher risk of going unmatched.

Realize there is no magic formula for ensuring you'll match where you want, or even if you'll match. But the advice offered in this chapter reflects multiple discussions with PDs across the nation, surveys of PD, and more than 30 years of experience. Good luck!

REFERENCE

1. Steven J. Weissbart, Soo Jeong Kim, Richard S. Feinn, and Jeffrey A. Stock (*2015*) Relationship Between the Number of Residency Applications and the Yearly Match Rate: Time to Start Thinking About an Application Limit?. Journal of Graduate Medical Education: March 2015, Vol. 7, No. 1, pp. 81-85.

For more information, please see the Medical Student Survival Guide *online at emra.org.*

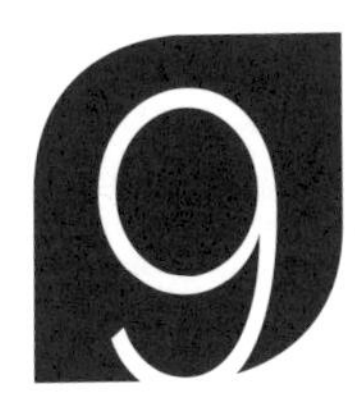

Surviving the Interview

Michael C. Bond, MD, FACEP, FAAEM
Associate Professor
Residency Program Director
Department of Emergency Medicine
University of Maryland School of Medicine

Amal Mattu, MD, FACEP, FAAEM
Professor
Vice Chairman of Education
Department of Emergency Medicine
University of Maryland School of Medicine

> *Scheduling interviews back to back can be very tiring, so give yourself some downtime.*

As emergency medicine residency positions become more competitive, the interview process has become an even more critical component of securing a preferred residency position. The process is additionally stressful since many graduating medical students have limited interviewing experience. Therefore, it is vitally important that applicants be well-prepared for the interview and represent themselves well during the entire process. This section will highlight pearls and pitfalls of the interview process.

Securing Interviews

One of the most stressful parts of the residency match process is obtaining interviews. In 2015, 2,352 applicants applied to the 171 EM residency programs that offered a total of 1,821 positions.[1] Therefore, the number of applicants exceeds the number of first-year residency positions in emergency medicine, and there are insufficient interview slots to accommodate all the applicants who apply to any given program. It is imperative that your ERAS application packet is as strong as possible and highlights all of your accomplishments to help ensure you get invitations to interview. Tips for maximizing the positive impact of your ERAS application are provided in Chapter 8.

The number of programs to which you apply should be based on the strength of your overall packet and presumed competitiveness. An experienced emergency medicine mentor will be able to provide more specific advice. In general, most applicants should apply to approximately 30 programs with the hope of securing 10-12 interviews, though this number can vary depending on the strength of the individual applicant. Ultimately, this number may need to be increased if you are attempting to match into different geographic regions, are part of a couples match, or if you have lower USMLE scores/rotation grades or other areas of concern in your application. Chapter 8 has additional information about choosing programs to apply to.

Scheduling the Interviews

Since the majority of interviews occur between November and January, arrange to be free of clinical requirements for at least one month during that time period, and preferably two, to allow you the flexibility to schedule your interviews. If you cannot be free of clinical rotations, make sure to schedule a rotation that will allow you ample time to travel for interviews.

Many residency programs are using services such as Interview Broker® that will send you an email with a token that permits you to schedule and reschedule (if needed) your interview by going to a central website. While this is convenient for everybody, it also means the most preferred interview slots go to those who respond the quickest to their emails. If the program is manually scheduling their interviews and you need to email or call them, it is critically important that you be cordial on the phone and have some flexibility in case your preferred date is already full.

Ideally, you will be able to schedule interviews in similar locations close together to reduce travel costs, but this is not always possible. Many residencies plan social events either the night before or the night of the interview. These social events are a great way to find out if you "click" with the residents and allow you to ask candid questions in a more relaxed environment. Allow time in your travel schedule to attend these events. Scheduling interviews back to back can also be very tiring, so try to give yourself some downtime between interviews so you remain energetic and upbeat. It is understandable to be tired if you have interviewed three days in a row, but the third program may see your tiredness as disinterest, which can affect your ranking in their program.

Your interview starts with your first contact with the program, whether by phone, an email, or the actual interview. This is your first impression, and it will have a lasting effect on your relationship with the program. Any interaction before, during, and after your interview day will be used to determine if you are a good fit. Assume that anybody you talk to in person, on the phone, or via email has a say on where you will be ranked. You definitely do not want to come across as demanding, cocky, or rude. Being polite, nice, understanding, and flexible will be remembered — and often the residency coordinators will bend over backwards to help you... but they can also break you! Poor phone etiquette or rudeness to a residency coordinator will almost certainly be discussed with the program director and will destroy your chances of matching at a given residency program.

Declining or Canceling Interviews

When interviews are initially offered, everybody grabs them up as quickly as possible. However, after you have 10-15 interviews (general recommendation for the average student) it is completely reasonable to decline or cancel an interview to a program you are not that interested in. Interviewing at a program you think is going to be really low on your rank list, no matter the reason, is not a good use of your time, the program's time, or your limited financial resources. Programs expect to have applicants decline and cancel interviews, and they greatly appreciate it if cancellations are done as early as possible. Cancelling early allows the program to offer the interview to another applicant who might be extremely appreciative of the opportunity. However, cancelling the day before or the day of the interview is not considerate of your fellow applicants or the program. Even worse is just not showing for an interview; this will often result in a phone call to your dean or home program director to inform them of this unprofessional behavior.

Therefore, cancelling or declining interviews is expected, especially with applicants being told to apply to larger and larger number of programs. Please just cancel or decline your interview as early as possible so another interested applicant can use the spot.

Preparing for Interviews

Preparation for the interviews starts with being an active member of the emergency medicine community. It is highly recommended that you become a member of one of the EM societies (AAEM, ACEP, EMRA, SAEM, etc.). As a member of one of these organizations you will start to receive journals, newsletters, and emails about the field. The newsletters will often highlight the latest challenges the field is facing. Reading these publications will help you speak more thoughtfully during your interviews and make it clear this is the field you want. EMRA also has many amazing resources on their website, along with other resources like this book, to help you through the interview process. For instance, EMRA has a residency interview guide available at http://bit.ly/1IAKm2m that provides more than 142 questions the programs might ask you and another 65 questions you might want to ask residents, faculty and program directors.

Most residency programs have well-developed websites that can provide a wealth of information about the program. Read their websites before you interview. Ideally, you'll review the sites even before applying to the program to make sure there is nothing that would prevent you from ranking them highly. Why waste your time interviewing at a place that you would not want to rank well? Having a basic understanding of the program (e.g., how many hospitals do they rotate through, are they a 3- or 4-year program, what elective opportunities do they offer, what benefits are provided) will allow you to ask pertinent questions and help show that you have a true interest in the program. It is also important to know the names of the key players are in the department (e.g., program director, chairman, etc).

The final step in preparing for the interview is to ensure that you have a business suit that fits and looks good. The color or style of the suit does not matter, but what does matter is that it is clean, professional appearing, and it is not distracting. A bright orange suit might look great in a club, but it will also make you very memorable, probably in the wrong way, during an interview. If you are planning to have multiple interviews in the same week it is best to have more than one outfit to allow time for dry cleaning, and to have a spare in case you spill something on it. It is very easy to change the look with a different shirt and tie or a different blouse, so a second complete suit is not necessary. For women, make sure you are wearing comfortable shoes and avoid very high heels, short skirts, and revealing blouses. The program directors are assuming this is the best you will be, the most professional you will ever look, and that you will be on your best behavior — so don't be anything less than what they expect.

The Interview Day

It is worth repeating: The Golden Rule is that "Program directors assume you will be the best they will ever see you on your interview day." PDs assume you are putting your best foot forward and will be on your best behavior, be well-groomed, polite, and courteous to all you meet. A conservative appearance is recommended. Though you want to show your true personality, the interview day is not the best time to have multicolored hair, multiple facial piercings, or to be flamboyantly dressed. The interviewer's imagination will start to picture how you will appear on your first shift if you are comfortable enough to show up on an interview day this way.

Remember that all your interactions are taken into account when the program decides where to rank you.

As previously stated, remember that all your interactions are taken into account when the program decides where to rank you. Avoid bad-mouthing other programs or getting into heated debates about politics or religion, even with the other applicants. Exchanging information about other programs is perfectly acceptable, as you will often see the same people on the interview trail, but you will never know who might know somebody at the other program, or worse, who trained at the program you are bad-mouthing.

Allow enough time to arrive at the interview a little early. All programs will provide an itinerary or tell you when to show up for the interview. Arriving 10-15 minutes early is acceptable, but arriving much earlier can be a burden on the residency staff. Often they are busy with last-minute preparations, and they will feel the need to entertain you. Wait in the building's lobby or in your car before heading up to the interview area.

Most interview days will start with an overview of the residency program, information on the local area, and other information the program feels would help you make a decision about their suitability for your training. The overview is often followed by several interviews. These can be done one-on-one with faculty or residents, or in a group setting. Some programs do standardized interviews, while others will have unstructured interviews. The programs can ask you about anything in your application, so if there is anything you are not comfortable talking about, do not include it. For instance, if your motivation for going into emergency medicine was because you witnessed the death of a family member, but you get emotional, tearful, and uncomfortable talking about it, then it is best not to include that story.

Be prepared to speak on any of the activities on your ERAS application, especially any publications or research you have done. You should have a good understanding of these areas. You should also be prepared to speak on areas of interest in emergency medicine. For example, two common questions are "What challenges do you anticipate having to overcome during your career?" and "How do you think the ACA is affecting emergency medical care?" Other common questions are "Do you have any ties to the area?" and "What will be your ultimate job once you are done with your training?"

During the interview it is recommended that you sit in the chair properly and lean forward slightly. Be careful not to lean too close to the interviewer so you are not violating his/her personal space. It is also recommended that you not recline in the chair, bounce it back and forth like a rocking chair, or lounge about. Finally, be mindful of your body language and any nervous habits (e.g., picking at your nails, twirling your hair, etc.).

When asked a question, take a moment to collect your thoughts and answer it directly. Try not to ramble, and ensure you have some pauses so the interviewer can ask another question or acknowledge what you have said. When given the opportunity, try to have some questions to ask about the program.

You should not be asked any questions about family planning (e.g., "Do you plan to have kids during residency?"), race, religion, national origin, ancestry, disability, marital status, or sexual orientation. However, if you bring up these topics during discussions or mention them in your application, including your personal statement, then the door is opened and the interviewers can discuss it with you. If you are uncomfortable discussing any of these topics, then it is best to just not bring them up. There is no standard way to deal with these questions if they are asked. Some people will answer, while others will deflect and answer a slightly different question or try to change the subject. It is up to you how you handle the situation and ultimately, whether you decide if this should affect how you rank the program.

The Tour and Social Event

The interview day almost always includes a tour of the hospital. The hospital tour is your opportunity to see the various parts of the hospital in which you will be working. For emergency medicine you will typically be shown the ED, intensive care units, and any medical floors where you might rotate. Use the tour as an opportunity to ask about support services (e.g., are there transporters, ECG techs, IV techs), nursing relationships, working relationships with off-service residents, and faculty-resident relationships. Remember the tour guide has an opinion on where you will be on the rank list, so be respectful and do not monopolize a single individual's time. You should also pay attention to the physical plant and its condition. Is the place in need of repairs, are they renovating, are there plans for expansion or renovations in the future, and is the place clean?

Similar questions can be asked during the social event. This is also a great time to ask about life in the city. Do the residents have any concerns about living in the area? Where do the residents live? Do they feel safe walking to their car or home? What is the cost of living? What do they do for fun or to relax? Do the residents hang out together?

Some residency's social events may include alcohol. It is perfectly acceptable to partake, but you don't want to be labeled as the "drunk" or the person who drank several pitchers. Moderation is key. Also have self-awareness of how alcohol affects you, and be careful if you are likely to lose your inhibitions and start talking too freely.

If you are not provided specific guidance on the dress code for the social events, plan for business causal.

End of the Interview

At the end of the interview season, many of the interviews will blur together and you will forget details that could affect your rank list. It is recommended that you take some time immediately after each interview day to sit in the lobby or your car and write down some notes about the program and hospital. Write down everything you liked or disliked about the program, or triggers that might help you remember your interview day. These notes will be very important when it comes time to rank the programs.

Thank-You Notes

It is good practice to send a thank-you email or letter to the program director. Some programs may tell you it is not required, but unless they tell you this we recommend that you send a short note thanking them for the interview. This is common courtesy and the norm for most occupations in our society. Most applicants also include a few personal comments thanking the interviewers for any career advice, for information about the city, or for taking the time to discuss specific topics of interest. Some PDs might use the thank-you note as a marker of your interest in their program, so it's advisable to send at least a brief note if you are interested in the program.

Follow Up

Many students ask about emailing the programs later in the interview session, especially if they interviewed early. They often fear that they might not be remembered as well as somebody who recently interviewed. Not to worry. The programs take extensive notes and will not forget you, but sending a late email can serve two purposes. The first is that it can show true interest in the program, as long as it is individualized and personalized to the program. Second, it can update the program on any other major accomplishments, USMLE results, or letters of recommendation that might have been entered after you interviewed. Do not send a mass email stating that you are really interested in 20 programs. There is also no need to tell a program you are ranking them highly. Most program directors take these comments with a grain of salt, as we all have had applicants tell us that and then match in another program.

Conclusions

The residency interview is a great opportunity to learn more about the program, ensure that program is a good fit for you, and give you an opportunity to learn about the city and hospital. While interviews can be stressful, some minor preparation (professional attire, learning about the program and the field of emergency medicine) can eliminate a lot of the stressors and make the interview a great fact finding experience. Just remember to always be your best. The rest will take care of itself.

PEARLS FOR SURVIVING THE INTERVIEW

- Research the residency program and be familiar with the program's leadership, structure, and educational opportunities. This will allow you to ask more specific questions to address your needs and show your interest in the program.
- Clean up your social media profile to ensure there are no damaging photos or posts out there. One site, www.socialsweepster.com, can automate the scan, even looking for telltale red Solo cups in your online photos.
- Dress professionally. Use appropriate language. Avoid slang or derogatory comments.
- Prepare an opening statement that highlights who you are and what your ultimate career goals are. This could be a quick summary of your personal statement.
- Stay focused on the presentations and interviews. Turn off your cellphone so you do not get distracted. If your wife is expecting, give them the phone number where you are interviewing instead of your mobile number. Nothing says "I am not interested in your program" more than you checking your phone during the interview.
- Send a thank-you note unless you are told the program does not want them. This can be done via email or regular mail.

REFERENCES

1. NRMP 2015 Main Residency Match Advanced Data Tables

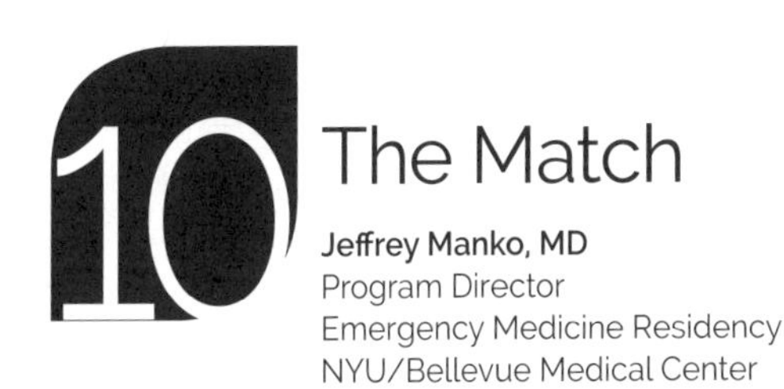

The Match

Jeffrey Manko, MD
Program Director
Emergency Medicine Residency
NYU/Bellevue Medical Center

Welcome to the process that represents the culmination of all your hard work in medical school: **THE MATCH**. Even the name gives the impression of a marriage or lifelong commitment that will change the rest of your life. However, once you understand the match, you will find it far less intimidating. This chapter is here to help you navigate through the intricacies and nuances of the match process.

What is The Match?

First, the match represents the coupling of medical training programs with prospective residents to form mutually beneficial relationships. Students apply for these training relationships — residencies — through ERAS, which is run by AAMC. The participating residency programs, meanwhile, are managed by the Accreditation Council for Graduate Medical Education. The National Residency Matching Program then matches students with programs, based on rank order lists from each party. So you apply through one organization for programs that are managed by a second organization, and a third organization actually handles the match.

> ***Once you understand the match process, you will find it far less intimidating.***

Applicants and programs each create a rank order list showing their preferences in candidates and programs. The NRMP rates applicants' rank lists ahead of programs' lists. (For an example of how it's run, visit www.nrmp.org/wp-content/uploads/2014/05/Run-A-Match.pdf.)

Clearly, a tremendous amount of time and energy is invested by both applicants and program directors into the match process. It is extremely important to understand that as much as you want to be happy with your choice, the program directors want you to be happy with your choice (and theirs) as well.

Emergency medicine as a specialty has been growing in popularity during the past decade, achieving a double-digit increase in residency positions, according to NRMP data. The number of students pursuing emergency medicine has risen, and so, too, has the number of emergency medicine programs and therefore emergency medicine spots. Currently, the ratio is close to 3:4 spots to applicants.

In 2015, there were 171 emergency medicine programs with 1,821 applicant spots for 2,352 PGY-1 applicants (1,613 U.S. seniors). The program fill rate was 99.6% with 8 spots being unfilled.[1] Although emergency medicine is very competitive, you should be optimistic about your chances of landing a residency spot.

Preparing for the Match

When deciding on a program to do your training, it is important to factor in many variables. The Accreditation Council for Graduate Medical Education-Residency Review Committee (ACGME-RRC) ensures that accredited programs meet standards to ensure you will be appropriately and adequately trained in emergency medicine to pass the ABEM certification exams. Emergency medicine has several program formats, ranging from 3- and 4-year programs to longer combined residencies (e.g., EM/internal medicine, EM/family medicine, EM/pediatrics, etc.), which only adds to the complexity of your decision-making. Rest assured all the formats train excellent emergency physicians. Whether you go to a small, rural program or a large, urban program, you will learn how to intubate, treat myocardial infarctions, reduce fractures, and other essential EM skills. The emergency medicine curriculum is similar in all programs, so you don't have to worry about lacking essential training.

This frees you to consider other factors — or "happy outside the hospital, happy inside the hospital." The idea is simple. If you are satisfied with your geographic location and your personal life, you are much more energetic and enthusiastic about your job. As residents you will spend an inordinate amount of time in the hospital (even with the duty hour guidelines), but you should take into consideration the things you like to do outside the hospital when thinking about programs where you might like to match.

Couples Match

All of these recommendations assume you are doing this solo. If, however, during the course of your medical education you have managed to find the love of your life who is also in the same boat, then you will need to consider entering the couple's match. The NRMP accommodates applicants who wish to be matched as a couple by allowing two individuals to form pairs of choices on their primary rank order lists, which are then considered in order of preference when the matching algorithm is run. [source: NRMP Results and Data 2015 Main Residency Match] So what does that actually mean? Well, the devil is in the details — but if you want a couples match, you can do it. In 2015, the NRMP received a record number of couples match requests, with a total of 1,035 couples participating. Couples enjoy great success, with a PGY-1 match rate of 94.8% [source: NRMP Results and Data 2015 Main Residency Match]. If you need details about the couples match, visit http://www.nrmp.org/match-process/couples-in-the-match.

Time to Apply

Applying to residency programs is streamlined with the Electronic Residency Application Service. All of your letters of recommendation (including SLOEs), the Medical Student Performance Evaluation (a.k.a. dean's letter), personal statement, curriculum vitae, transcripts, and USMLE scores are uploaded to the same site to be retrieved by whichever programs you designate. Just a click of a button (and a little more money), and you can apply to as many programs as you can afford. Speak to advisers, current residents, and former students to help narrow the field to those programs you might actually be interested in. There is no penalty to applying to programs that you feel may be a "reach" based on your medical school academic performance, but it is critically important to be realistic about how competitive an applicant you are. Applying to only the most competitive and top-rated programs when you have a marginal transcript and below-average board scores would not be considered realistic.

The Interview

After your application is complete, all the supporting letters are in ERAS, the boxes have been clicked, and the fees have been paid, you will find yourself checking your email incessantly, waiting for the invitations to interview. Then, the responses start to arrive, and your whirlwind tour of the United States will begin. Take some time now to re-evaluate where you want to live and how much money you have budgeted for travel. Try to group your interviews geographically to cut down on flying expenses (unless you need to accumulate a boatload of frequent flier miles). To cut down on lodging expenses, look up old friends and distant relatives for a spot in the guestroom or on the couch. You may also be offering your couch to a college friend who is interviewing in your city.

Hopefully you receive many interview invitations. You do not have to go to every program that invites you, but you do have to show proper etiquette and withdraw your application in a timely manner if you decline. It shows a complete lack of courtesy and respect when applicants simply do not show up for a scheduled interview. DO NOT DO THAT! Someone on the waiting list would have gladly taken that spot to interview. A call in advance is expected and always appreciated by the program. If there are unforeseen circumstances (e.g., weather, traffic, illness), make sure you let the program coordinators know or leave a message as soon as possible to see if your interview can be rescheduled.

Making Your Rank Order List

After all your interviews are completed and your bank account is depleted, it is time to sit down and make your "rank list." Some important recommendations:

1. Rank the programs according to your preference (based on whatever criteria you choose to use). Your No. 1 program should be the one you would MOST like to attend, even if you consider it to be a "reach."

2. Where you think a program will rank you should have NO bearing on where you rank the program. Assume you are at the top of everyone's list and make your list accordingly.
3. Rank ALL the programs you would be willing to attend. A program may not be your first choice, but you should still rank it, if it is one you would not mind matching at (better than not matching at all).
4. NEVER rank a program you absolutely do not want to attend.
5. The match is BINDING for both the applicants and the residency programs. Make your decisions accordingly.
6. Expressions of love and devotion between applicants and programs are NOT binding and NOT commitments. (If I only had a dollar for each time an applicant told me I was "number one" and then s/he matched elsewhere...)

Speak with the important people in your life. Decide on your priorities and preferences, and make your list. After the list has been entered into the system and certified, the waiting game begins. Unlike when you applied to college and medical school, and you waited by the door for each school's acceptance or rejection letter, there is only "Match Day." One day in mid-March, all senior medical students around the country (and world) will receive an envelope with only their matched program listed inside. Congratulations, and hopefully you are happy with the results!

If You Don't Match

If you unfortunately do not match, you will be notified a few days earlier than the official Match Day, and you will enter the Supplemental Offer and Acceptance Program (SOAP). This process, facilitated by NRMP, takes place during Match Week and involves several rounds of attempting to pair unmatched candidates with unfilled residency spots. If you find out you didn't match, you should hear from your dean's office right away, but the most important thing you can do is to stay calm, keep a clear head and understand the SOAP process. While your dean's office is going to be very interested in helping you find a match, remember that you're not their only concern, so you'll need to make sure you follow all the rules and meet all the SOAP deadlines yourself. More information about the SOAP process can be found in Chapter 11.

Hopefully, this has provided you with some tips on how to approach the match. This is an exciting time as you embark on your career in emergency medicine. There are a growing number of emergency medicine programs available across the country, and the fun is finding the one that is just right for you. Good luck on this adventure, and I look forward to having you join me as a member of this exciting specialty.

REFERENCES

1. NRMP 2015 Main Residency Match Advanced Data Tables

Life After The Match

Colleen A. Crowe, MD, MPH
Assistant Professor, Associate Program Director
Medical College of Wisconsin

Alicia Pilarski, DO
Assistant Professor, Assistant Program Director
Medical College of Wisconsin

After Match Week is over, you are left with essentially two possibilities: 1. You have matched into a residency program, or 2. You did not match into a program. In either case, the next several months will bring significant life changes, both personally and professionally.

You've Matched...What Now?

Matching into a residency program can bring a whirlwind of emotions. No matter what you are feeling, your classmates are going through the same experience. Take time to discuss this new chapter of life with your colleagues and friends. Celebrate with people who will be joining you on your new journey (significant others, spouses, children, families, friends). If you are disappointed with where you matched, talk with your adviser or mentor who can help you make the best out of a situation that may not be ideal. Always remember, residency is only a short few years, so making the most of your situation is in your best interest as you work to become an educated, caring, well-rounded, and respected emergency physician.

Finishing Fourth Year

Typically, most MSIIIs will already have the second half of fourth-year rotations and electives established. If you haven't already figured out your schedule for the remainder of your fourth year, consider doing rotations in specialties that will help you become a more well-rounded emergency medicine physician. If you feel particularly weak in one area of medicine that you know you will encounter in the emergency department, seek more experience in that field. Some examples of rotations that are helpful for a new EM resident include ophthalmology (learning how to use a slit lamp and doing a good eye exam), ENT (managing epistaxis), dermatology (differentiating between benign and serious rashes, general management and understanding of common rashes), radiology (master reading a chest x-ray and other plain films and learn basics of CT scan anatomy), or neurology (perfect your neurologic exam, understand the differential of a "dizzy" patient). Another option is to do an elective in something you have always been interested in but didn't have time for, such as an international medicine elective, a rotation with a medical examiner, research, wilderness medicine, or any other subset of medicine that you find interesting and exciting.

Preparing for Your Residency

If you are moving to a new city or state for your residency program, the most important thing will be finding a place to live. Talking with current residents in the program, visiting the area, and researching the various neighborhoods are very important in determining the right place for you. Several factors come into play with this decision. Are you moving alone or with a significant other or family? Do you want to live close to the hospital for an easy commute? Do you prefer outdoors or city life to enjoy on your days off? Discuss safe neighborhoods with current residents, and also find out where current residents live. If you are moving with a significant other, be sure to keep his/her needs in mind. You will be spending a lot of time in the hospital, and want your family to be happy!

Although it is tempting to buy something, consider that residency is only a few years, and having a house to take care of in addition to your busy residency schedule could be an extra challenge — not to mention expense. Consider waiting until you have found a job after residency to purchase that dream home.

Moving can be a challenge in itself. Most programs have some activities at the end of June (welcome events, social gatherings, and sometimes orientations), so find out and plan accordingly. Depending on the size of the move (cross country vs. across town, house vs. an apartment, moving yourself vs. moving a family), you may want to consider hiring a moving company.

Another question that is always asked of residency directors is "What should I study before I start residency?" Consider that you have been studying for residency your entire medical school career. Depending on experience and background, some people may be more comfortable with the transition to a resident physician than others. Most medical students have little experience with writing prescriptions and dosages of medications. Reviewing common medications used in the ED (e.g., pain medications, anti-nausea medications, antibiotics, ACLS drugs), their indications, dosages, and side effects can be helpful for your first day on the job. If you feel particularly weak in any other specific area of emergency medicine, you may want to review some basic concepts. But rest assured you will get the training you need to succeed as an emergency medicine physician through your residency program.

Wrapping Up Your Fourth Year

After the Match, life will seem to move even faster than ever before. New experiences, possibly new locations, new friends, new mentors and teachers, and new responsibilities will be on the horizon. However, remember those who supported you through the past four years of medical school. Acknowledge and appreciate your current teachers and mentors, and seek any additional advice from them before you move on to your new role as a resident. The final few months of medical school tend to be less busy and more flexible, so prioritize time with family and friends, since free time in residency tends to be even scarcer than in medical school. Take a trip somewhere you have always wanted to visit. Plan dinners out with friends from medical school. Organize special outings or events to celebrate your new journey into residency. Time in the last few months of medical school should be used to its fullest. Re-energize yourself, get sleep, read something non-medical, or do something that will help bring you back to being who you are so you are ready and roaring to go come July 1.

You Didn't Match: Now What?

You've worked tremendously hard throughout medical school, decided on a specialty you thought would make you happy, and now you're told you didn't match. This can be an emotionally devastating time, but it is your job to take control of the situation. You didn't get your first choice — but that doesn't have to be the only choice.

The most important question to ask yourself: Are you absolutely set on a future in emergency medicine?

- If yes, then consider exploring the SOAP process to see if there are any unmatched EM programs. Or consider doing a transitional year (also achieved through the SOAP process) and apply again to EM next year.
- If no, what other fields held your interest? Consider exploring the SOAP for unfilled positions in another field that once captured your interest.

SOAP: The Nuts and Bolts

On Monday of Match Week, you will learn *if* you matched. If not, one option for you is to enter the Supplemental Offer and Acceptance Program managed through ERAS. SOAP runs through a series of rounds starting at 2 p.m. ET on Monday and concluding at 5 p.m. ET on Thursday of Match Week. During this time, you will be able to access the list of unfilled programs for any positions in which you are eligible. You are not allowed to apply to or contact programs outside of ERAS, nor should others contact programs on your behalf.

This is not a challenge to face on your own. Reach out to your dean's office — they have likely led students through the process in the past and are there to help you. In addition, talk with your adviser, EM clerkship director, or other EM mentors with whom you feel comfortable. They also may have advised previous students in the same situation. A key lesson in emergency medicine is to know when to ask for help — this is one of those times.

Whether you choose to pursue an open EM position or an unfilled spot in another field (or perhaps you choose to apply to a combination), you will submit your ERAS application to any and all areas in which you are truly interested in matching. If there is ever a time to be honest with yourself, this is it. Be both open-minded and realistic.

Programs will subsequently create a preference list in what is called the "R3 system" (***Registration, Ranking, and Results).*** A program can only make offers based on the number of unfilled positions. For instance, if a program has 10 residency slots and only matched 7, that program can make 3 offers during the first round of the SOAP. If one of the offers is accepted by an applicant, and the other two offers are rejected, that program will then have 2 unfilled positions and therefore can make 2 offers during the subsequent round. Bottom line: there are a lot of applications to a few positions and programs can only make a limited number of offers.

Applicants can receive *multiple* offers in any round and will have 2 hours to accept or reject an offer. This is where you need to remain realistic. Your heart was set on EM and during that first round of the SOAP you get an offer from an amazing program in your second-choice specialty. Offers that are rejected or expire (after 2 hours, when the round ends) will not be extended again. There are many applicants for only a few positions. At the same time, unless your first-choice offer appears, do not accept too quickly — you have the full 2 hours to await offers. Stay calm and focused. Most important, know that an accepted offer is a binding agreement. Once accepted, you are committed to that residency position.

The SOAP Didn't Work

Perhaps the SOAP process isn't successful (there are no open EM spots, the SOAP process didn't result in your favor, or you chose not to go through the SOAP). There are some other options.

a. Extend medical school. Some medical schools will allow you to stay on for a 5th year and reapply to residency. Inquire with your medical school, and be sure to understand the financial implications. In some cases, you may be able to obtain another degree (i.e. MPH), do some research, or simply gain more clinical experience. If you opt for this choice, it is important that you tailor your schedule to augment your EM application. Do more EM rotations (and ace them!) both at your home institution and away. Try to get clinical rotations that are particularly beneficial to a future in EM (e.g., trauma surgery, critical care, radiology, etc.). If there was a particular area of weakness on your application, this may be your chance to show improvement. Seek advice from EM faculty mentors on how to improve your application.
b. Research. This is another option to utilize some of your skills while filling the gap of time before reapplying to residency. Note, however, that EM residencies will want to see continued clinical experience. If at all possible, try to obtain some clinical rotations or at the very least, clinical shadowing.

This can be a very challenging time — a time to remain humble and ask for guidance from your mentors who know you best.

The authors would like to thank *Larisa Coldebella, MD, Thomas Grawey, DO* and *John Pokorney, MD.* for contributing to this chapter.

Financial Advice for the Future Emergency Physician

James M. Dahle, MD, FACEP
Department Chair, Utah Emergency Specialists
Founder, The White Coat Investor website
Author, *The White Coat Investor: A Doctor's Guide to Personal Finance and Investing*

> ***When you find yourself deep in a hole, stop digging.***

I joined EMRA as an MSIII in 2001 or so, and shortly thereafter came into contact with the first edition of The EMRA Medical Student Survival Guide. It definitely affected my career and my life for the better, so I feel honored to be able to give back to the guide to help those who are now entering the specialty. However, that original edition did not include anything like this chapter. Most of the knowledge in this chapter I obtained in the school of hard knocks throughout medical school, residency, and my first decade as an attending. Consider the sharing of this advice, along with my own financial mistakes and successes, a personal gift to you.

The Most Important Year of Your Life

Most of you reading this chapter will be MSIIIs, MSIVs, or interns. There is very little you can do at this point in life to improve your financial position. There are a few minor things I will cover later in this chapter. However, the most important thing you can do financially at this stage is to prepare for what will be the most important year of your life, at least financially speaking: the year you graduate from residency. You see, it is easy to overcome most of the financial mistakes you make as a resident, simply because your income grows you out of them. That is not the case once you are an attending.

Consider an emergency physician I once met at a conference where I spoke on financial topics such as those in this chapter. He was in his early sixties, making about $300,000 per year, and had a net worth of $300,000. While that might sound like a lot of money to an MSIV, the truth is that physician at that point in life should have had a net worth closer to 10 times that amount, and possibly even been retired already. He had probably earned $5-$10 million in his life, and all that was left was a measly $300,000, despite having decades to save and let compound interest work on his savings. "Where had all the money gone?," I had to wonder. The truth was most of it simply had been spent, although a significant portion had been lost in poor investments. If you follow the simple, but not necessarily easy, directions in the next paragraph, you will never be in this situation.

The secret to eventually being the wealthy physician your family and friends think you are is to live a lifestyle very similar to your resident lifestyle for the first 2-5 years after residency. If a resident is making and living on $50,000 per year, and then his/her income increases to $300,000 per year (about the average for emergency physicians in a recent salary survey), there is a $250,000 per year difference. Some of that, perhaps $50,000-$75,000 per year, will go to taxes. However, that still leaves $175,000-$200,000 per year with which to build wealth by paying off student loans, saving up a down payment for a house, and maximizing contributions to retirement accounts. Most doctors (and especially their spouse or significant other) will be unable to completely resist the temptation to grow into their new income. But even if the doctor gives herself a "50% raise" and lives on $75,000 per year, there will still be at least $150,000 per year available to use for wealth building. Even a high student loan debt burden, such as the $300,000-$400,000 many residents now graduate with, won't last long against an assault of that magnitude.

What the doctor cannot do, however, is buy the big house her partners have, drive a nice car like her partners have, go on the expensive vacations her partners go on, cut back to 10 shifts a month like some of her partners might have, and basically live "a doctor's life." Not yet. That day will come, and if the doctor will live like a resident for just a few years, it will come much sooner than she thinks.

How do I know this works? Because I did it for about 4 years after residency. By the time I had been out of residency for 7 years I lived in a fancy "doctor house" that was 1/3 paid for, I had no student loan burden, and I had a net worth of over $1 million. And I did it on an average salary of around $180,000. It wasn't complicated, and there is no reason you cannot do the same. I no longer "live like a resident," although I am still frugal relative to my income. I am still in my 30s as I write this, yet have retirement and college savings essentially already paid for and am practicing emergency medicine on my own terms. I could work 6 shifts a month for the rest of my life if I so chose. Night shifts are optional for me. If I were fired, I could literally go years without working without having to worry about how I was going to feed the mouths at my table. If you also want to be financially independent, live like a resident for 2-5 years after residency. That is the most important financial advice any physician can be given.

Your Second Job

Most physicians, and frankly most people, have not yet realized the world has changed. Everybody now has a second job — as a retirement portfolio manager. Previous generations benefitted from the existence of pension plans. You did your 20 or 30 years for a single employer, and then they gave you a gold watch and paid you a monthly income from the date of your retirement until the day you died. Now, in our "401(k) world" we are all expected to know how to manage our own retirement pension, despite never having received any formal training in doing so. You will need to get this training on your own or find a competent, low-cost adviser to assist you with the task. Don't worry, it is far less complicated than nephrology or even figuring out how to work up and treat pulmonary emboli. You need to implement a system of "Continuing Financial Education" (CFE) beginning early in your career. Medical school and residency are times to focus on learning how to practice medicine to the very best of your ability. However, there is still time to begin the CFE process. I suggest you follow a good financial blog and read at least one good finance or investing book per year.

Living Well Below Your Means

Most people know of the importance of living within your means. What they don't realize is that if you merely live within your means, you will never acquire any significant wealth. The key to doing that is to live not only below your means, but well below your means. Although new attendings should live like a resident for a few years after residency, they will eventually be able to loosen the purse strings significantly. However, I still recommend that you save around 20% of your income at that point. Although you might not be able to save quite that much as a resident, I suggest instilling this habit from your very first paycheck as an intern. Remember that as hard as it might seem to live on just $50,000, there is somebody down the street living on just $45,000 per year. Live like him and bank the difference.

The transition from living on student loans to living on earned income is a difficult one for many medical students. Having $200,000-$400,000 of student loan debt can make you numb to what that really means. It is so scary that residents are often in denial as to its consequences on life 5, 10, or even 20 years down the road. Do not let the fact that you have a seemingly insurmountable debt hanging over your head confuse you about the need to live within your current income. Your eventual attending income will allow you to escape that debt, but not if you keep digging during and after residency. When you find yourself deep in a hole, stop digging. Don't take out additional loans to live on or even to go on job interviews. When you make your residency rank list, be sure to factor in the cost of living in that locale. Living frugally is a bit like building muscle. The more you practice, the easier it becomes and the stronger you get. Start practicing with your first paycheck.

Manage Your Student Loans Properly

Tuition bills have soared. To make matters worse, despite record low interest rates everywhere else in the economy, student loan interest rates have remained high. But wait, there's more. Now professional student loans aren't even subsidized ("subsidized" loans mean the government pays the interest while you are in school). These factors cannot be ignored. If you do not have a plan to get rid of your student loans rapidly, you may wake up one day in your late 50s and realize you still owe thousands for classes you took over two decades ago. However, the news is not all bad. There are three good things that have happened with student loans in the past decade.

Many physicians can have a good chunk of their debt forgiven.

The first is the lower payments available to residents through the Pay As You Earn (PAYE) program, which is similar to Income Based Repayment and Income-Contingent Repayment, all outlined by the Office of the U.S. Department of Education at https://studentaid.ed.gov/sa/repay-loans/understand/plans/income-driven. Each of these programs is slightly different, but the bottom line is the payments you make in residency are based solely off your income, rather than the amount you owe or the interest rate of the debt. While this has the unfortunate effect for most residents that their debt actually grows during residency despite making payments, the truth is that most residents can't afford to make real payments on their student loans anyway. A debtor with a $400,000, 7%, 10-year student loan has annual payments greater than a resident salary.

The second bit of good news is that many physicians can have a good chunk of their debt forgiven. The best forgiveness program is the Public Service Loan Forgiveness program. After you have made 120 qualifying payments while employed by a nonprofit hospital or a government entity, the remainder of your debt is forgiven, tax-free. If you made 36 or more tiny PAYE payments while in training, there is likely to be a 6-figure amount still to forgive. In fact, it is possible for a physician to have more forgiven than s/he ever borrowed. Most residency and fellowship programs are qualifying employers. Most academic positions are as well. Many nonprofit hospitals also offer direct employment that will qualify, but merely working for a private group that contracts with a nonprofit hospital does not qualify. There is also forgiveness available through the PAYE program, but it requires 240 total monthly payments, and the forgiveness is taxable. This is not a good option for most emergency physicians, as most will have their debt completely paid off in less than 20 years.

The most recent good news is that in 2015 it was possible to refinance student loans with private companies at rates in the 2%-5% range. Medical students and residents probably should not refinance their loans as they need the lower PAYE payments and do not yet know if they will be working for a PSLF-qualifying employer. Companies won't refinance most residents anyway. But upon residency completion, if a doctor is not going to be working for a PSLF-qualifying employer, s/he should refinance student loans and then live like a resident until they are paid off. Some medical students and residents are afraid the government may change the terms of this program before they receive their promised forgiveness. Just in case, payments equivalent to student loan payments should be made into an investment account. That way, if the forgiveness fails to materialize, you can liquidate the investments and still be free of your debt burden within a few years of residency graduation.

Protect Your Most Valuable Asset

The most valuable asset a physician has is his/her ability to earn a living. Over the course of a career, a typical emergency physician will likely earn between $5-$20 million. Until you are financially independent (do not have to work to support yourself and your family) you need to have sufficient disability insurance in place. Life insurance is simple, because life is pretty black and white. As an emergency physician, you're familiar with a few grays areas there, but within a few hours, it's all going to be sorted out when it comes to death. Disability, however, is 50 shades of gray. Because of that, disability insurance contracts are complicated. Independently purchased contracts are the most likely to pay you in the event that your disability falls into one of the gray areas (such as mental illness, substance abuse, chronic pain, vague neurologic or rheumatologic conditions, etc.). They are also more likely to pay you when you are only partially disabled, when you are returning to work, or when you have income from another source. Independent policies are also portable, in that they can be taken with you when you change jobs. However, group disability contracts provided by your employer are likely dramatically cheaper. There is no right answer as to what type of policy or policies you should get, and which features you should pay for. The bottom line is that you ought to have something in place. I suggest you meet with a good independent insurance agent who can sell you specialty-specific policies. Compare the features of any group policy you may qualify for with those available from individual disability companies and make an informed decision. Disability insurance is expensive (expect to pay 2%-5% of the income protected each month) but never more critical than early in your career.

If you have people depending on you, such as a spouse or children, you also need to have life insurance in place. The type you want is "term life" rather than a "whole life" product, which is lifelong insurance policy combined with an investment account with a low return, neither of which most physicians need, and certainly no resident needs. Purchase either a 20- or 30-year level term policy (where you pay the same price every year until the term expires) or an annually renewable policy. The benefits of the annually renewable policy are that you can purchase more insurance with the same amount of money when you need it most but can least afford it (as a resident and young attending), and that if you become financially independent in fewer than 20-30 years and drop the policy you will have significant savings. The downside, of course, is that the premiums go up each year and may become unaffordable while you still need the insurance. As a general rule, early in your career, your insurance face amount should be measured in millions, not hundreds of thousands. A healthy 30-year-old female can get a $1 million, 30-year level term life insurance policy for around $50 a month. An annually renewable policy may be as little as a third of that price.

Should You Buy or Rent Your House In Residency?

There is an interesting, and almost universal, phenomenon among graduating medical students, especially if they are married with children. They want to buy a house and view renting as a terribly inferior alternative. The truth of the matter is that the default option for most residents should be to rent their home during residency. Are there exceptions? Of course. Buying a house does work out better than renting in some circumstances, but they are far rarer than most graduating doctors believe. I have had to make the "buy vs. rent" decision 5 separate times in my married life. Three of the 5 times I made the decision incorrectly, once because I did not understand everything that should have gone into the decision, and twice mostly out of pure bad luck. In all 3 situations, it cost money that to me was significant at the time. Luckily, I eventually do learn, and when it came time to spend the big bucks, I had the experience to make the decision correctly. I will go through several myths that cause inexperienced buyers to make these decisions incorrectly.

Myth #1: Renting means living in an apartment.

In most areas and in most time periods, you can rent a house that is just as nice as you can purchase.

Myth #2: If I rent, I can't make the changes I want to make to my house.

Most landlords would be overjoyed if you wanted to do some home improvements and add some paint. They are likely to furnish the materials if you will furnish the labor. They won't let you knock out a wall or paint the house some terrible shade of purple, but the truth is if you want to sell a house you own anytime soon, you can't do that anyway.

Myth #3: If I sell the house for more than I bought it for, then I will come out ahead.

Most inexperienced purchasers fail to understand just how expensive it is to buy and sell property. A good general rule is that you will spend 5% of the value of the property when you buy, and 10% when you sell. The realtor fees alone when selling are 6%. However, you are likely to have to do some upgrades, pay for closing costs for the purchaser, and do repairs that turn up during the inspection. The house might sit empty for a few months between the time you move out and the time it is sold, costing you more money. The expenses upon purchasing are often rolled into the loan, but they exist nonetheless. Thus, in order to come out ahead, and all else being equal, your house must appreciate by more than the transaction costs. If the house appreciates at 3% (never a guarantee), and you have 15% in round-trip transaction costs, then you will need to own the house at least 5 years just to break even. Emergency medicine residency only lasts 3-4 years, and most residents are leaving town upon graduation. Even those who stay aren't likely to want to stay in their "resident house" for long.

To make matters worse, appreciation does not happen in a straight line. There are periods of time, such as 2003-2006 when I was renting during residency in Tucson, when property appreciates dramatically. There are other periods of time, such as when I lived in a townhome as a young attending from 2006-2010 (the housing bubble crash) when property depreciates dramatically. After 9 years, that home is still worth slightly less than I paid for it. The real estate market can be difficult to time, but consider where you are in the housing cycle when making the buy vs. rent decision. If property is sitting for months before being sold at fire sale prices to investors, then it may be a great time to buy. If you find yourself in a bidding war with other purchasers, consider renting. Holding a property for 10 or 20 years will allow you to spread the transaction costs out over enough years that appreciation will be a bigger factor. But if you are only going to be in a house for 3-5 years, luck will be a much bigger factor in whether or not you make money than you think.

Myth #4: If the mortgage payment is less than rent, then I will come out ahead.

Real estate investors know there are far more expenses involved in owning a property than just the mortgage. These include fire insurance, flood insurance, earthquake insurance, taxes, repairs, maintenance, property management fees, HOA fees, snow removal, and lawn care. Renters generally do not pay any of these. Thus, in order for a real estate investor to have positive cash flow (i.e., make money each month), the rent charged must cover not only the mortgage, but also all of these other expenses PLUS leave something for profit. Thus, a mortgage payment SHOULD be dramatically lower than the rent payment on a comparable property. I made this mistake on a condo I bought in medical school. Rent and the mortgage payment were comparable, but I never factored in all of the other costs that would be involved. Although I sold it for slightly more than I paid for it, I came out way behind after transaction costs.

If, despite these warnings, you do decide to purchase, there are a couple of things that can help improve your returns. The first is to use a "doctor mortgage" that allows you, for slightly higher fees and a slightly higher interest rate, to put little to nothing down without having to pay Private Mortgage Insurance (PMI),which is insurance lenders make you purchase to protect them if you default on your loan. There is no benefit to you.

The second is to look into government down payment assistance programs designed for low and middle income families. It is not uncommon for a resident to qualify for $10,000 in free money, which can obviously sway the buy vs. rent calculation significantly.

Getting Started Investing

As you learn more about personal finance, you will find yourself wanting to get started investing. It is important that physicians, even residents, understand how their available retirement accounts work. Your employer may provide a 401(k) or 403(b) to you. Read the provided plan document. Understand the investment options and the associated fees. Determine if your employer will match your retirement savings. If so, be sure to contribute enough to the account to get the entire match. Not doing so is the equivalent of leaving part of your salary on the table. Determine if there is a "Roth 401(k) or Roth 403(b)" option (meaning you pay taxes on the money when you earn it, but not when you withdraw it from the account decades from now). If there is a Roth option, be sure to use it in residency while you are still in a low tax bracket. If there is no match, you should do any investing you do inside a personal and/or spousal Roth IRA. You can contribute $5,500 from your income to each of those accounts each year. Once you become an attending, you can continue to make Roth IRA contributions, but due to some odd tax laws, these contributions must be made "through the backdoor" utilizing a Roth conversion. If you choose to moonlight as an independent contractor during residency (and wish to put away more money toward retirement,) you can open an "individual 401(k)" and make additional retirement contributions there.

Be sure your investments are low-cost and broadly diversified.

No matter what investment account you use, be sure your investments are low-cost and broadly diversified. I suggest using index funds from a company such as Vanguard. You can buy index funds that invest in U.S. stocks, international stocks, bonds, and even real estate. If you are unsure what to invest in, one of the best default options is the Vanguard Life Strategy Moderate Growth mutual fund. When you purchase shares in that fund, you will essentially be buying all of the stocks and bonds in the world at a very low cost. At this stage in life, the return on your portfolio matters far less than your savings rate. Earning an extra 2% on a $5,000 portfolio is only $100 a year. Eating out one fewer time each month could make a difference six times that large.

You will not be able to save and invest much as a resident compared to when you become an attending, but establishing good habits early, and giving compound interest as much time as possible to work, will literally pay great dividends.

Learn the Business of Emergency Medicine

During medical school and residency, you will have some exposure to emergency medicine as a business. This won't, and probably shouldn't, seem very important to you as a trainee, but there will be a day when it matters to you much more. Take advantage of any available opportunities to learn about coding, billing, business structures, contracts, and the various types of employment arrangements. Whether you choose to be an independent contractor doing locum tenens, a partner in a small democratic or large democratic group, an employee of a Contract Management Group (CMG), or a hospital or university employee may have a dramatic difference on how much you are paid and how much control you have over your work. Always remember the general rule that a business owner cannot pay you 100% of what you are worth, or there will be no profit coming out of the business for the owner. The only way for you to get that 100% is to own the business yourself, with all the responsibility that entails.

You are embarking on a wonderful career where you will make a real difference in the lives of some of your patients and co-workers. However, it is not without its downsides. Burnout in emergency medicine is very real. The best antidote to it is to never feel like you HAVE to practice emergency medicine. If your finances are in order, you can practice on your own terms. This will make you a happier person, a better spouse, a more loving parent, and a more competent and compassionate doctor. Feel free to contact me with any questions at editor@whitecoatinvestor.com.

REFERENCES

http://www.amazon.com/The-White-Coat-Investor-Investing/dp/0991433106

http://whitecoatinvestor.com/financial-survival-guide-for-new-interns

http://astore.amazon.com/whicoainv-20?_encoding=UTF8&node=70 (Book Recommendations)

http://whitecoatinvestor.com/personal-finance/the-doctor-mortgage-loan

http://whitecoatinvestor.com/disability-insurance-introduction

http://whitecoatinvestor.com/10-reasons-why-residents-shouldnt-buy-a-house

http://whitecoatinvestor.com/how-to-buy-life-insurance

http://whitecoatinvestor.com/backdoor-roth-ira-tutorial